# MORE METHOD

THE SIMPLE FORMULA TO GET **MORE** OF EVERYTHING YOU DESIRE IN LIFE

JEN GROOVER

**The MORE Method**



Published in the United States by Change Her Story, Inc

Change Her Story
1703 N McMullen Booth Road
#201
Safety Harbor, FL 34695



ISBN 13: 978-1-951781-00-2

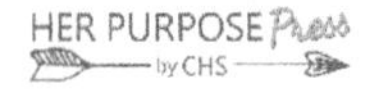

# Praise for The MORE Method

*"If you're feeling stuck or limited and you know you're capable of more...but you just don't know where to start...you need Jen Groover's, The More Method! At a time I needed it most, The More Method provided me the tangible strategies to gain clarity, confidence and momentum in my business. My personal growth - without question - surpassed any other personal development book, course or program I've experienced. If you want to more in your life - personally or professionally - Jen Groover'sThe More Method will undoubtedly change the trajectory of your success beyond what you may ever expect!"*

**Lindsay Vastola**

Founder, VastPotential Leadership Development

*To say that Jen Groover's MORE Method presentation was amazing would be a grave understatement. We are so grateful for her bringing The MORE Method to Toll Brothers. It has positively impacted and improved all of our lives.*

**Andrea Ferrino**

Media Manager, Toll Brothers

*Jen Groover has been a mentor of mine for many years. Her MORE Method strategies have increased my self-awareness and made me the leader I am today. Jen lends her experiences from her personal and career stories to teach lessons on empathy, compassion and gratitude; ultimately how to be your best self to have the best life. Her success is proof that leading from the heart and understanding people can cultivate happiness and profits.*

**Alex Grant**

Mindset Coach and Former NCAA Gymnast

*Learning from Jen and The MORE Method principles has been life changing! She helped me get to the root of many of my self limiting beliefs, taught me how to reframe my thoughts and to manifest a better life for myself, both personally and professionally. Jen gives you the motivation and tools to transform your life, live joyously and grow beyond measure. As a direct result of Jen's coaching and guidance, I was able to accomplish my goal of becoming a speaker and a bestselling author. I am forever grateful for to tools she has given me. I know this book will help you achieve your goals and live the life you desire too!*

**Amy Banocy**

Entrepreneur, Speaker, Author

*Jen Groover's approach to helping individuals and teams become more self-aware, confident and emotionally intelligent to succeed at new levels is amazing. She articulates perspectives in an engaging way with simple yet powerful insights. What is needed for improvement quickly becomes apparent, achievable and exciting. Those who actively engage in the concepts find more fulfillment and productivity as individuals, professional teams, and even families. I highly recommend reading her book and working with her to help everyone reach their potential!*

**Matt Stephenson**
Executive Vice President, Rogue Credit Union

*Meeting Jen Groover was the catalyst to my success. As a mentor, coach, trusted advisor and now friend, she has changed my life. The MORE Method helped me to challenge myself and gave me the tools and confidence I needed to overcome my limited beliefs. Thank you Jen for writing this book!*

**Professor Theresa M Agostinelli**
Certified Executive Coach, Speaker,
Leadership Trainer, Licensed Psychotherapist

# DEDICATION

This book is dedicated to anyone I have met throughout my life journey — from young to now — you have helped shape me; through good experiences and painful ones; whether friends, family, acquaintances, or just passerbys, I thank you. For each experience has helped me learn and grow, and created content that I am able to share today to help others.

For my daughters, who are my greatest teachers daily. I am grateful you have so willingly "shared" me with the world throughout your lives to help others. Thank you for continuously inspiring me to be the best person I can be, to be the best example I can for you.

For my mother and father who are no longer here today, I thank you for doing the best you could with what you knew and what you went through. I am grateful things were the way they were so I could use the lessons to passionately do this work I love so much and help others break cycles.

For anyone who believes we can consistently evolve and become better versions of ourselves, but wants more tools to evolve faster, this book is for you.

# CONTENTS

# INTRODUCTION

If you have this book in your hands, I am more than grateful for your time and trust in me with what I am about to share with you.

I know time is our most precious commodity so I am always conscious not to waste it; for myself or others. I always have a clear intention to be adding value to the lives I have the ability to connect with. So here is my **MORE Promise** to you for spending time with me.

This book is intended to take you on a journey of self-discovery and transformation to continuously become your best version self, to create your best life possible.

When you read AND engage with the exercises in this book, The MORE Method will teach you to:

- Become more heightened in your self-awareness
- Have more clarity to create the life you desire
- Identify more of the beliefs and behaviors that block you from getting what you desire
- Create more fulfilling relationships
- Have more energy and mental clarity
- Develop more effective communication skills
- Become a more intentional creator
- Learn how to see life from multiple perspectives
- Have more confidence and greater sense of self worth
- Connect more deeply with other
- Create more empowering daily habits to thrive
- Have more inner-peace and be less affected by others around you
- Have more wholistic success
- Live left with more gratitude and intrinsic happiness

- Create a more fulfilling life that you love
- **BE MORE OF YOUR BEST VERSION OF SELF**

...and so much more!

I am excited to take you on this journey and look forward to hearing from you after you are finished this book.

Much appreciation,

Jen Groover

# The MORE Method DECLARATION

**I believe** that every person can change, evolve, and improve—no matter their stage or age of life.

**I believe** that people stay stuck, stagnant, or in many repetitive destructive cycles simply because they don't know what they don't know.

**I believe** most people never come close to accessing their potential because they have been conditioned to do the minimum to get by.

**I believe** that most have never realized how much greater life can be, in all aspects, when we become the most expansive version of ourselves.

**I believe** the reason most people settle for so much less than what they are destined for is because they never knew how to get MORE of everything they desire out of life or believed that they were worthy or capable of having a better life.

**I believe** that if people are given the proper tools to change and improve, they can – but only if they desire to.

*It is my life's mission to teach anyone, from any age, from any background, from any season of life, how to get more of everything they desire in life.*

## CHAPTER 1

# Be **MORE** to Achieve and Receive **MORE**.

My dysfunctional childhood was a training ground for everything I teach. I understand trauma, pain, abuse (in many forms), fighting, divorce, scarcity, manipulation, sick parents, and dying parents. But I also understand joy, happiness, success, love, inner peace, fulfillment, inspiration, empowerment, and beautiful relationships — and what it takes to get there.

I never allowed my childhood to limit or define me. I chose to let it inspire me for MORE and I let it teach me about duality and contrast. **There is so much power in contrast; learning about what you don't want helps you to find clarity as to what you do want**.

I call these our **MORE Moment Stories**— the moments in your life when things are less than ideal to motivate you to transform your future.

Before we dive into the MORE method, I want to tell you a little about where I come from.

One of my first childhood memories was watching my dad throw my mom down a flight of stairs. Her head hit the basement floor and blood began to pool around her. My brother and I were at the top of the stairs, looking under a locked door.

I was 4 years old, my brother was 5.

My mother had taught my brother how to dial "0" (911 didn't exist back then) if an emergency happened and he had memorized our address. In that moment of panic, my brother took action, which probably saved my mom's life.

My dad was a highly functioning alcoholic at the time. He would start drinking after work with his colleagues at the local bar near his office, and most nights he came home drunk. On the weekends, we were always at parties or places with a bar.

Dad was the really fun guy once he got going, but inevitably, there was a tipping point from the fun (numbed) guy to the angry drunk. That is when the abuse would set in. Many nights, we slept in the back of our station wagon or would flee to safety at the homes of friends and family.

These types of early childhood experiences were very stressful and often traumatic, but were an important factor to who I became and why this book exists today.

*Before I go any further, I want to be clear about something really important—probably one of the most profound lessons of this book: I do not harbor any ill will toward my father and these early childhood experiences. I have chosen to see these experiences as gifts that taught me pivotal lessons.*

*My father recently passed away and I am so grateful we were at peace in our relationship, or I imagine the experience could be a lot more psychologically disruptive than losing a parent already is.*

**My dad did his best with**
**the tools that he had.**

*He grew up in an emotionally unavailable environment, and the conditions around him led the way to where his future life journey would go. At that time, men did not seek "help" to be better versions of themselves like many men do today. They were considered "successful" if they provided financially for their family. When there was trauma or dysfunction, it was numbed or swept it under the proverbial rug as if whatever the problem was simply didn't exist. Being vulnerable or emotionally available was not seen as a "manly" trait.*

*I made peace with all of my difficult memories by giving them meanings that helped me make sense of the events in a positive way. By assigning them positive meaning, I was able to fill these memories with compassion and empathy instead of anger. Understanding this concept is fundamental, as well as one of the fastest ways to break bad cycles and create MORE of everything good in your life.*

My mom was a strong, sassy woman from Brooklyn. She was an early model for Seventeen Magazine and met my dad in Philadelphia while on a photo shoot. A hair straightening product had caused my mom's hair to fall out, and my dad—an attorney at the DA's office at the time—represented her. That's when they fell in love.

Mom was different from the women my dad had met before. Her strength was attractive to him... until it wasn't. She came from an old-school, intact Italian family. My grandparents were the stereotypical "Frank and Millie" Italian couple, and Mom worshiped her father because he was so sweet and loving. They spent time together often, and went to as many baseball and football games as possible. Mom grew up to be strong and empowered.

My dad grew up poor and with emotionally unavailable parents. He joined the Marines, and eventually put himself through law school and became a successful attorney and Magistrate. He taught me important skills and work ethic. It was from him that I learned that you get nothing until you earn it. He always emphasized the importance of determination and pride from accomplishment.

The first years of their marriage was a whirlwind. Dad was charismatic and charming when he wanted to be. Despite knowing he had a problem, Mom found herself in love with a man who would strap her on a permanent rollercoaster.

The day of my first clear childhood memory—when my brother saved my mom—was just the beginning of years of rollercoaster rides for my brother and me, too. And although my father eventually got sober, the pain and anger remained for years. During those stressful times of my childhood, I still had some valuable experiences that exposed me to the goodness of life and the possibility that the future could be your own creation.

Though my mom suffered in her own home, she did many exciting things professionally and took my brother and I with her when she did. She ran campaigns for politicians and believed in active participation. She believed in being a voice, not just a vote. I spent many hours of my life in campaign headquarters, pep rallies, door to door campaigning, and watching victory speeches. I was always in awe of the energy and the "bigness" of it all. We hated being dragged around at the time, but I believe seeing her in action shaped who I am.

She also had an award-winning television show for Cablevision called "For You and About You" about current affairs. Because of her love for sports, she often had professional athletes join her on the show. Legends like Steve Carlton, Tug McGraw, and Ron Jaworski graced her stage. If you guessed I'm from Philly, you'd be right.

My brother and I often sat in the studio after school. At the time, I was resentful because I wanted to be outside playing with my friends. But I realize now how profound of an impact my afterschool studio time had on who I am today. We listened to interviews with many high-level thinking and achieving people—so many pearls of wisdom seeping into my impressionable brain.

Looking back on that time, I can now see that I also had great self-preservation skills. I learned how to "escape" stressful moments by diving into my imagination and spent hours with my friends. Ironically, all of my good friends had intact, supportive families who treated me like family. I was invited to many dinners, sleepovers, and family vacations. While I had a stressful home life, I also saw how different things could be through the lives of my friends.

In college, I studied education and psychology (which it seemed many people with crazy childhoods did). In my first class, I learned about positive reinforcement and it blew my mind. I was in awe of the fact that I didn't really need to be hit with belts and wooden spoons to be a good kid. I was shocked that there was a better way to enforce rules— ways my parents clearly didn't know about.

The more I learned about psychology, the more I was obsessed with this thought: "Why on earth aren't these courses mandatory for everyone? The world would be a better place if everyone would learn what I was learning!" For the first time in my life I was excited about school. I was passionate and connected to what I was learning. It was a clear tipping point to my future.

During one holiday break when I was in college, I took one of my days at home to visit the local gym. That day, I attended my first step aerobics class and I loved every second of it. Loud music, fun choreography, and a room filled with high-energy people made an hour workout feel like 10 minutes. I was hooked. Having been an athlete, most of my experience of "working out" revolved around activities that made you feel nauseous afterward. But this just made me feel vibrant and alive. I knew I needed to continue it when I went back to school. So, I figured out how to get certified and helped create a group fitness program for my university. I didn't realize it yet, but this was the first of my entrepreneurial experiences. Every time I taught a class, I felt so alive and high on life. It was a sensation that I savored and would continue to seek as the state I wanted to be in the majority of my life.

Once I decided I wanted to dive into the fitness industry full-time, the universe helped align amazing opportunities. I had a bartending gig a few nights a week at that time, and as luck would have it, I ran into a guy I knew. He had attended a neighboring high school to mine and was also in the fitness industry. After chatting a bit—with me gushing about my fitness industry aspirations—I found out that he was a partner in a gym. He and his business partner were looking for a woman to help attract female clients and start a group fitness program. And bam! My life began to accelerate from there.

Fast forward to a few years later; I had become a National Level Fitness Competitor. I was a master trainer and traveled all over, preaching the power of being fit. You'd think I was an expert in fitness, right? Well, as it turns out, I was over-exercising and not resting enough. While on the outside I looked like the essence of "fit", I was falling apart on the inside. My kidneys, liver, heart and thyroid all were affected. I felt exhausted all the time, no matter how much I slept. I felt passionless, which was the opposite of how I wanted fitness to make me feel. I began to feel depressed and withdrawn. But no one on the outside would have known, because I constantly forced on a smile and drank enough caffeine to keep moving.

After searching for a couple years to figure out what was wrong, I found out that I had oxidative stress. I had also developed multiple autoimmune suppression issues, including Hashimoto's Disease.

Remember how I said I look at difficult experiences as gifts to teach me? The gift from that time was that I was becoming more and more spiritually awakened in my quest to get out of my struggle. Again, I believe the Universe provides all the tools you need around you. If you can see them, you can use them. I could have been a victim, but instead I chose to just figure out how to get better and evolve from the experience. Looking back, I realize I had so many clients who were providing resources for me from their own struggles. Books they were reading, I began reading. Workshops they were going to, I attended. And the conversations they were focused on became some of my favorite kind of conversations. They were deep conversations around the meaning and purpose of life. This type of spiritual discovery helped me heal, not just physically, but also emotionally from my childhood wounds.

Thankfully this happened when it did, because it laid a powerful foundation for the experiences that were about to transpire in the years that were ahead of me.

In 2001, I was married to a wonderful soul who created the first real sense of stability in my life, especially in my home sector. And, in 2004, I gave birth to twin girls. Had I not been so persistent in getting to the root of my health problems in the years before, there is a good chance my girls wouldn't be here today.

I am always fascinated with how many "sliding doors" occur in our lives, where one seemingly small thing can change the entire course of one's life. Although I have come to expect miracle moments like that, they still always fascinate me.

I was never really the girl who was the 'babysitter" growing up, so going from having no children to two children at once was quite a transitional challenge. It came with a great sense of joy, but it was overwhelming at the same time. There were so many new skills I needed to learn, and there were many things that were programmed into me during my childhood that I did not want to bring forward into my daughters' lives.

**If we are unaware of our childhood programming, especially the things we**

**don't like, we will likely subconsciously program those things into the next generation.**

I was determined not to do that. This forced me to dive even deeper into my personal and spiritual growth.

When my daughters were 3, my mother passed away, along with quite a few other significant people in my life—all within a three-month span. My mother's passing shook my world in a way I never expected. It was like opening a Pandora's box of all of my unhealed childhood mess. A floodgate of questions and confusion surfaced. The biggest realization I came to was that we can't shove issues under the proverbial rug, because they will always come back. The longer we avoid them, the harder life will become. Although I was extremely self-aware at this point, the universe was making me go deeper. To the deepest points possible. My spiritual quest and desire to understand myself and the meaning of life deepened even more.

The Universe kept providing the right people and experiences to help guide me to become who I am today, sharing with you this book. I believe there are lessons and opportunities for growth in every single experience of our lives. The problem is, most of us aren't looking for these opportunities. We are not even present enough to see them right in front of our faces. Most people go through life continually wasting these gifts, then complain about how they can never catch a break. Some even complain that the world is against them and how they have bad luck. **Their mindset just continues to create the experiences they are perpetuating with their beliefs.**

A few years later, I found myself going through a divorce. And although it was the most amicable situation possible, it shook up my world in a profound way. It rattled my first grounded "home" experience and made me go even deeper in my healing and awakening. As this transition began, my greatest intentions were to 1) learn to love at my greatest capacity like I had never experienced before; and 2) heal and continuously reveal my greatest self.

When you ask something BIG like this of the Universe, it will deliver—but not usually in the beautiful, picturesque way we think we want. Instead, to get BIG results like this you will have to go through some messy, painful experiences that will make you want to quit— but I am sure glad I didn't.

I think it's important to mention that throughout this entire journey, from my first business in the fitness industry until today, I always had mentors to help guide me through every step of my life journey. They were their cheering me on or, even better, calling me out on my stuff in those moments that I did feel like giving up. Mentors and coaches are vital in any aspect of life you are trying to improve upon.

As I continued to heal, evolve, and transform, I took careful inventory of what was helping me the most so that I could share it with others. (That eventually led to the book you are holding in your hands today.)

This book is the culmination of my 20-plus years of teaching human potential. As I evolved, my content and teaching have evolved, and will continue to evolve. At my core, I have always loved learning, assessing, and then taking my knowledge and turning it into wisdom to share with others who are ready to learn. All of these lessons have created new tools in my toolbox that I want to share with as many people as possible.

**The more effective tools we have, the better we can construct our lives.**

The MORE Method came to me in the middle of the night many years ago with lightning-bolt-like clarity. Before I went to bed, I challenged myself with a deep question: What separates you from everyone else in your industry? What REAL value are you bringing to everyone's lives? What's the key thing you do for everyone?

I woke up to a clear message saying, "You teach anyone, at any stage, how to get MORE of what they desire in life. You provide simplification of big ideas and theories and help people make small changes that have a big impact." With complete certainty, I realized the value I could give others was the MORE Method. Then, within seconds, the breakdown of the acronym MORE became very clear, which you will be learning more about very soon.

## THE MORE METHOD

**M** indfulness in everything you do

**O** ptimization of body and brain

**R** esponsive versus reactive lifestyle

**E** xcelling in every aspect of life

**The teachings that I am sharing with you in this book have not only helped transform and optimize my life, but the lives of millions of others. I have no doubt it will give you useful insights and wisdom to level-up any aspect of your life you are seeking to optimize.**

I have written this in a way that you can easily highlight, reflect, journal, discuss, and execute. I believe you will get the most out of this book by participating in the journaling exercises provided throughout the book. So before we get started, begin by grabbing your MORE Method Journal.

Once you have completed the exercises in this book, go back and re-read your MORE Method Journal dozens of times, because as you evolve, so will what you are taking from the content here.

As I mentioned earlier, this method brings several disciplines together to create a simple formula of how to get MORE of everything you desire in life. I am excited to begin the journey now with you!

## Journaling Prompts

1) What do you hope to achieve by reading this book and completing the journaling exercises? What desires are on your mind and heart?

2) What memories and experiences maintain a negative hold on your life? How can you use those experiences to seek positive outcomes?

3) What accessible tools do you see around you? These can be physical objects, places, experiences, motivations, people, or anything else you observe in your surroundings.

4) What ideas, values, and perspectives were programmed into you during your childhood? Which of these things are you eager to pass on to the next generation, and which do you want to actively avoid passing on?

## CHAPTER 2

# The **FOUNDATION**

## Clarity. Believe. Remove. Create. Repeat.

I have often wondered why so many people choose to complain about their lives rather than celebrating more of the good things every day. I find myself baffled because so many intelligent people miss the chance to live a fulfilling life in exchange for a life stuck in a loop—especially since most do not have to.

This mindset comes from years of being programmed to believe that a safe zone is what we need. It may have started with an adult who meant well in your life—one in a place of influence who said, "Oh, don't dream that big, I don't want you to get your hopes up!" For most of us, *this* is where the programming to diminish what we are capable and worthy of having begins.

**The truth is, if we never let ourselves dream or desire, we have already lost.**

When we don't allow ourselves to believe or even attempt to follow our desires and passions, we let the fear win.

Much of our society operates on this fear-based system which was projected on us unintentionally from previous generations. In trying to be helpful, they were sometimes ignorant of the power of the mind and manifestation. But this notion that life is better in the safe zone is a plague to our society. This plague robs people of their dreams, passions, love, and fulfillment, and shields people from recognizing their own amazing potential.

I once heard a life-changing quote from Erma Bombeck: "When I stand before God at the end of my life, I would hope that I would not have a single bit of talent left, and could say, 'I used everything that you gave me.'" You can suspend religious affiliations from this statement, and still acknowledge its power. Can you say this is how you are living your life today?

**You are worthy and capable of having what you desire in life. It is possible.**

**GROWTH is what derives happiness.**

The journey to being the best version of yourself is the gift. When you shift your mindset to value the journey, you will lose the fears of the discoveries you'll make and attachment to the destination to make you happy or whole. When you seek your greatest awareness, you will become who you need to be for something beautiful to happen in your life. Often these are not even things you expect, but are more amazing then you imagined. But that cannot happen in your safe zone.

I feel it's important to clarify here that when I say, "you can have what you desire in life," I don't necessarily mean living a life in which you amass great financial fortune and materials. It could mean that to some people, which is totally fine—but what I really mean by playing to win is that you wake up on a regular basis living a life you have intentionally created. A life you feel grateful and blessed to be living. A life that you find to be meaningful. A life that you feel happy and at peace in most of the time.

I understand that some of life's circumstances are not always ideal. However, you will learn in this book that even when things aren't ideal, we always have the power to give circumstances meaning that can turn pain into purpose.

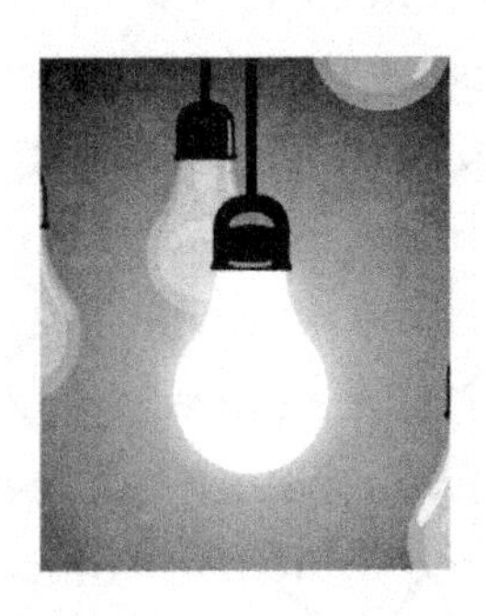

**ENVISION** what you want

**BELIEVE** you are worthy and capable of having it

**REMOVE** the beliefs and behaviors that keep you from it

**INTENTIONALLY** take action and create the life you desire

## To get MORE of whatever you desire in life you must:

**Step 1)** Get a **CLEAR** vision of what you really desire and why.

**Step 2)** **BELIEVE** you are worthy and capable of your desires.

**Step 3)** **REMOVE** the beliefs and behaviors that are currently blocking you from what you desire.

**Step 4)** Become a daily **INTENTIONAL** creator, making more conscious choices that support your desires.

## Get a Clear Vision of What You Desire

As I mentioned earlier, so many of us have gone through life afraid to clearly envision what we desire because we fear being disappointed. Today I give you permission to let go of that fear and reprogram your brain with a belief that is more empowering. For example, instead of saying that you can't let yourself dream, say this:

**I can get MORE of everything good in life once I become more clear as to what I desire.**

Please take out your MORE Method Journal and a pen and begin to write down your list—*without editing in your head!* Do not limit this list. What do you want more of? What do you currently desire for your life? What do you find yourself daydreaming about and wishing your life would look like?

I know that if you are a goal-oriented reader, you may have done exercises like this before. Or maybe you have been encouraged to do exercises like this at work, where the list is mostly focused on external things like sales goals you want to meet. But I would like you to encourage you to approach this a little more holistically, starting from the inside out.

For example, coming from a stressful childhood, one of the things I wanted MORE of from life was inner peace. Consistent inner peace is one of my greatest accomplishments, but I never could have accomplished that if I didn't:

1) Become deeply introspective and clear as to what I desired most and why, which included envisioning what that could look and feel like

2) Believe I was worthy and capable of having it

3) Remove beliefs and behaviors that blocked me from my inner-peace—for example, if I held a belief like, "life is always going to be

hard and stressful," then I would act out those behaviors when interacting with others, seek validation of that belief, and never find my place of inner peace

4) Intentionally create a life that was calmer and more centered to make space for the life I desired—which included making conscious choices. One way I did this was intentionally distancing myself from people who caused drama and/or were constantly negative.

In the famous words of Mahatma Gandhi: "Be the change you wish to see in the world."

**This is an opportunity to BECOME what it is you desire from the inside out.**

As a mentor to many entrepreneurs, my clients often ask me to teach them how to build a million-dollar company. My response is always the same: "If you want a million-dollar company, you need to become a million-dollar person." When we become a person who thinks and acts like a million dollar person— abundant-minded, embracing creativity, emotionally connecting with people, letting go of fears, desiring to constantly make impact, giving back—it is easier to achieve the things needed to accomplish that goal and keep growing further (all while being happy).

If what you desire is a deeply loving, fulfilling relationship that is filled with vulnerability and rich communication, you need to become that person who is deeply emotionally available, open to love, not afraid to be vulnerable and a great communicator, instead of defensive, guarded and always waiting for the other person to disappoint you.

If you desire more thriving health and mental clarity, perhaps you need to become the person who is more grounded, prioritizes self-care and proper sleep habits, chooses more high-quality food, and chooses to be active over being complacent.

**Becoming what it is we desire is how we get MORE of what we desire.**

**So what is it that YOU want MORE of?**

Here are some suggestions from "the inside out"

- Self-love
- Love in your heart
- Inner-peace
- Joy
- Meaning
- Fulfillment
- Passion
- Confidence
- Spiritual connection
- Thriving health
- Increased energy
- Emotional harmony

- Feeling of safety
- Mental clarity
- Impact on others
- Positive perspectives
- Happiness and laughter
- Fulfilling relationships
- Harmonious loving family
- Satisfied customers
- Career fulfillment
- Financial security
- Material status

**Please note:** the list above has a domino-effect. The MORE you find what is on the top of the list, the MORE you naturally gain the things toward the bottom of the list. However, most people seek the things on the bottom of the list (like materials) to make them happier, more lovable, more confident, etc.

The mistake that we make (thanks to very skilled marketers in our world) is that if you gain more material assets, you will feel more of the things at the top, like joy, inner-peace, confidence, etc. That might be one of the biggest, most common lies that destroys the happiness of our generation. We desire external things (i.e. materials, job status, and relationship status) because we believe that in having them, we will be happier. So then why not seek authentic happiness first?

I am not saying that desiring material things is bad, but I am saying that desiring material things with the goal of feeling happier, more confident, and more loved is a complete illusion that leads to higher rates of depression, disappointment, and disconnectedness.

I suggest keeping your list nearby. Consider copying it onto a sticky note or notebook page and leave it somewhere you will see it every day, like your bathroom mirror or your refrigerator. Since it's easy to fall back into old patterns, frequently evaluate whether you continue to intentionally work toward achieving those desires.

## Believe You Are Worthy and Capable

Now that we have clarified what MORE you desire from life, you must believe that you are worthy and capable of having it. This may be a hard one depending on how you view yourself. But the most important thing you should remember is this:

**YOU ARE WORTHY AND CAPABLE BEYOND WHAT YOU EVEN REALIZE.**

I believe we are all worthy and everyone is here for a reason.

There is proven power in repeating affirmations to program new beliefs into our brains. This takes frequency, consistency, and conviction. Frequency and consistency are important to override the old programming. For example, if someone throughout your childhood told you that you were not worthy 1000 times, you should repeat that you ARE worthy a minimum of 1000 times. Ideally, you should repeat it at least twice as much. So much so that it just becomes who you are in your new mindset.

Start considering the affirmations that you need to hear. If you're not sure what to say, you can repeat my statement from above: "You are worthy and capable beyond what you realize." It may be more meaningful for you to craft your own affirmations based on your personal needs. What truths about yourself do you need to hear? If you want inspiration for something a bit more in-depth, here is my personal affirmation:

Conviction is extremely important, because if you say it without believing it or mumble through it without passion, you will not gain much from this exercise. Look in the mirror and repeat your affirmation every day. Envision what you want your life to look like and feel the power of the emotion of how it feels, as if it has already become, knowing you are worthy and capable of having it.

**Think of your body like a magic wand, attracting whatever you're affirming.**

I promise that this is a powerful exercise that will add value to your day. It is also an exercise that every thought leader I have studied under or observed will attest was a fundamental part of their transformation.

**In your MORE Method Journal, write down the affirmations that will begin to transform your future. You can also voice record them on your phone and listen to them in your own voice as you say them every day. This is even more powerful!**

## Remove the Beliefs and Behaviors That Are Blocking You

I am going to let you in on a huge secret I discovered from working in the human potential field for over 20 years. When I realized this pattern, it was one of those mind-blowing, ah-ha moments that I wished I had known from the beginning of life.

You ready for it?

**Whatever outcome you are currently experiencing in your life that you do not like or**

**desire, there is a belief attached to it that MUST change in order for you to get what you desire.**

Read it over and over again and let it really sink in.

I love uncovering patterns because once you discover patterns and their roots, it becomes easier to break the ones you don't want. This one was one of my favorite discoveries because it felt like I just unlocked the door to accelerated freedom. I found a way to free myself from my own self-sabotage.

I have worked very closely with people for a long time to help them remove patterns that no longer serve them, and it has become somewhat intuitive. My clients often joke that they think I am psychic because I am consistently able to spot their patterns. However, my greater desire is to give my clients the tools to uncover these patterns on their own.

Belief patterns have always been somewhat challenging to teach others because so many of our beliefs are so deeply ingrained in us that they are intertwined in how we view the world. Some beliefs are so deeply rooted in our subconscious mind that we struggle to even access them, even though they can be running (and maybe even ruining) our lives.

I call this phenomenon **Belief Blind Spots**. These are the pesky beliefs we hold onto that are more challenging to see and uncover—even if we desperately desire to deal with them head- on.

With this in mind, I ask you: What outcomes do you currently have in your life that you do not like and want to change?

Write them down in your MORE Method Journal.

Now, let's dive into these outcomes to find their root origins.

Let's think of the negative outcomes in your life like weeds. Have you ever tried to get rid of a weed by mowing over it or ripping the stem off of it? That will get rid of the unsightly blemish in your garden, but it won't get rid of the weed. The roots will remain, choking out the other plants in your garden from underground. And before you know it, the prickly leaves will grow back even stronger than before. What you need to do to get rid of a weed for good is dig deep enough to find its root. Once you've exposed the root, you can prevent the weed from growing back. And best of all, you can choose to plant a lovely flower in the hole where the weed once was.

What does that mean for your life? It means we can't just try to stop the negative outcomes on the surface; we need to dig deep enough to find the root origins of the negative outcomes in your life so we can stop them from growing. Only then can you replace that unwanted outcome with something beneficial.

Look back to the list of unwanted outcomes you wrote in your MORE Method Journal. Choose one and begin asking more questions to figure out the beliefs that have influenced that outcome in your life. For example, if you notice that one of them concerns money and work, begin to ask yourself things like:

- What are my beliefs on money?
- What are my beliefs on success?
- What are my beliefs on power?
- What are my beliefs on living financially free?
- What are my beliefs on going to the next level in my career?

Once you dissect questions like this around the core topic, peel back another layer.

For example, for the question: What are my beliefs on money?

Perhaps your answers are:

- It's hard to come by.
- It's the root of all evil.

- The people I grew up with won't like me if I have too much of it.
- You can't have a lot of it if you didn't graduate from a great college.
- You can't have a lot of it if you don't work really, really hard to get it.
- You can't have a lot of it if you aren't really smart.

Now, peel back again to try to identify where that belief came from:

For example: Where did I learn that money is hard to come by?

Believe it or not, not everyone believes that—and I assure you the people who believe it's easy to come by have an abundance of it. And you might say, "Well Jen, it's been hard to come by my whole life, so it's the truth." I would then challenge you to understand that what we believe, we attract. What we believe, our ego seeks for validation.

**And what we believe will continue to exist in our reality until we change the belief.**

So yes, if you were programmed throughout your childhood to believe that money is hard to come by and everyone in your community was living the same reality (evidence), and then as you got older you naturally surrounded yourself with people who believed the same thing (more evidence) and then you began your career and it was always hard to get ahead and have enough money (more evidence), you would believe that this belief is "truth."

But reverse engineer it: Because you believe it, is has become/been your truth.

Now you need to **change the belief** if it is no longer the reality you would like to exist. For example: Money is abundant everywhere and it is available to me because I am doing things to add value to the lives of others. This could become an affirmation for many.

Choose a statement that feels realistic to you. Then, start reading books and watching movies about successful people who you want to be like. Watch videos they have created. Listen to the conscious language they use. Observe their lifestyle and envision yourself as part of that lifestyle. Feel how it feels. Listen to mindset training audios/videos around abundance programming and meditations.

Lastly, (but very important) spend time with people who think abundantly and create distance with people who live from a place of scarcity. This isn't to say you should abandon everyone from your previous and current lives. But you should seek out people who are in the same headspace as you want to be in, and be selective as to who you let into your inner circle. You become the sum of the five people you surround yourself most. Be careful who you allow to share your space and influence you. Also be careful of who you allow into your social media feed, because that also becomes our reality.

It is helpful to have mentors, coaches and/or accountability partners who heighten your awareness and hold you accountable. They will be able to see things you may not see and hear things you don't even realize you are saying.

It is so easy to fall back into old patterns and beliefs that if we do not implement this strategy, it can be much more challenging to make consistent forward moving progress.

Once you finish mapping out how to change that belief, go back to your list of beliefs, identify the source of the next belief of the list, decide whether you need to change that belief, and map how you will move forward to make that change. (In this example, the next belief is "Money is the root of all evil.")

Once you finish mapping that list, go back to the previous list: the list of questions you asked yourself about one of your unwanted outcomes. Answer that question with the same method: provide several answers to the question and peel back the layers until you can identify where those beliefs came from. (In this example, the next question is "What are my beliefs on success?") Cycle through all of the questions you listed, peeling back the layers until you get to the root of how you came to the beliefs causing the unwanted outcome. Then map out any changes you need to make in the same way you did with the previous question. It will take a while, but don't rush. I promise it's worth it.

After you've completed a deep analysis of all of the questions you asked yourself, the answers, the sources of those answers, and any changes you need to make, move on to the next unwanted outcome you listed and repeat the process. By doing this for each outcome you want to change, you can begin to attack the weeds at their roots and decide what new beliefs you need to plant in order to reap the outcomes you desire.

These are the areas where people struggle the most:

- Money
- Power
- Relationships
- Health and vitality

- Age
- Integrity
- Truth vs. lies
- Personal development

## Intentionally Create the Life You Desire

How many days do you go through life feeling like you are flying by the seat of your pants? Or like your life is one big tornado chaotically spinning in and out of days without any time or energy to gain grounding?

The answer for most people to those questions is constantly.

But the truth is that it doesn't have to be like that.

We can become intentional creators. **Intentional creators are extremely aware of who they are, where they are, and where they want to go.** They are mindful of making conscious choices to move toward what they desire, even if it's the harder choice or delays gratification. Intentional creators pause more often, reflect, and plan throughout their days.

Once we become more intentional creators, our days feel more organized, more meaningful, and more productive. Better yet, we get MORE out of each experience. It is possible with just a few small pauses and tweaks in our schedule.

**There is so much power in our pauses**. But the sad thing is that people think they are "too busy" to pause. To that I say: "You are too busy NOT to pause." Being intentional with time is vital.

Here are a few tips to simplify becoming an intentional creator.

1) Make your schedule for your day the night before or first thing in the morning. If you are someone who is always late, wake up 15 minutes earlier. Those 15 minutes are worth so much more at the end of your day. As you plan out all the things you need to do, time block them.

2) Evaluate and reflect on why you are doing what you are doing. What are the intentions for each meeting? Imagine how many hours could be saved and how much productivity could be increased if everyone was clear in their goals and intentions for each meeting before they entered. This isn't just for business, this includes meetings/outings with family members and friends.

3) Assess who you are allowing to influence you. What are your intentions with who you spend your free time with? How do you

spend your free time? Do you consistently clarify your intentions to others to engage with you more effectively?

4) Ask this question constantly: is there a better or more efficient way to do what I am doing? Is how I am living my life supportive of working toward my goals?

5) Reserve moments in your day to pause and reflect on how your day is going. Could you have done something better? If so, how? This is something that is useful to journal about at the end of the day as you become more mindful of being more intentional. This skill allows us to course correct behaviors we want to change more quickly.

6) Start your day out with your daily affirmation and visualization practice. This reminds you of where you are going and helps continuously remind you to align your actions with your desires. Many, including myself, continuously do their affirmation and visualization practice throughout their days. This amplifies the clarity and energy

around where you are going and the choices needed to get there.

The process of intentional creation is powerful. It makes us feel more in control of how our life is going and creates space for a strategy of constant improvement when needed. This is a fundamental to the process of becoming the best version of ourselves.

Once you have mastered this phase, you can continue the next phase to get MORE out of life.

## Journaling Prompts

1) Look back at the list of things you want MORE of that you wrote in your MORE Method Journal. When you wrote the list, I asked you not to edit the ideas in your head. What did you write down that you would have edited out had I not asked you not to? What ideas came to your mind that surprised you?

2) If you had the power to completely reconstruct your life from this point forward, what would it look like? How would it be different from your current life? How would it remain the same? Consider your personality, your spirituality, your health, your career, your relationships, your free time, etc.

3) Turn back to the list on page 11. Which of these desires resonate with you most?

4) Reread the personal affirmations you wrote in your MORE Method Journal. How do you feel when you imagine realizing your desires, knowing that those affirmations are true?

5) What can you start doing this week to put into action the mapping you did to change your

beliefs and their negative outcomes? What can you do today?

6) When you sought the origins of your root beliefs, did you notice a pattern of where those beliefs came from? How might those common sources affect other areas of your life that you hadn't considered?

7) Where can you find people who have the mindset that you are trying to attain? What places might you go? What communities might you join?

8) At what points in your day can you schedule an intentional pause to assess your progress toward the life you desire?

9) How do you anticipate that the practices outlined in this chapter will put you on the path toward your best life? Which practices do you believe will be most helpful? How do you think these activities will affect your everyday life?

CHAPTER 3

# MINDFULNESS

## In All That You Do

Mindfulness is the foundation of all growth, transformation, and evolution.

**Having a solid awareness to who we are now is critical to who we can become.**

If you want a house to weather storms, you need a solid foundation. We invest and take so much more interest in making sure the external house we live in is stable, but all too often, we build our internal houses on unstable ground because we don't have the guidance on how to lay the foundation properly. Then, when storms come (as they always will), the houses without solid foundations fall. Some rebuild, some don't. The ones who rebuild have learned from previous experiences how to create a more solid foundation the second time around.

Storms can be profound moments of growth for those who seek wisdom and gifts from them. They can challenge us to rise and become stronger and more powerful.

But we can only embrace the challenges if we are mindful.

Mindfulness is a heightened sense of awareness in all aspects of our lives. I think of it as a process where we can step outside of ourselves and see a spotlight on how our life is going.

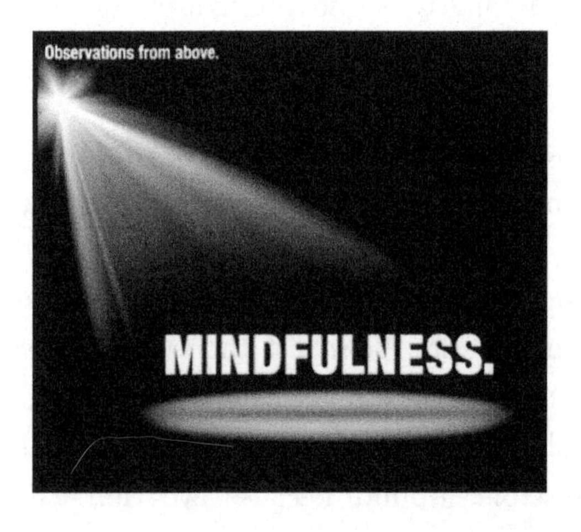

Mindfulness is what helps us master living a more responsive life instead of reactive life, which creates greater inner-peace, happiness, and fulfillment. The more mindful we become, the more we realize that we are in control of how we view the world and our circumstances. Even better, mindfulness allows us to live a more conscious path, make better choices, and have the ability to course correct faster when we get off track.

When we can become more masterful in our mindfulness, we become like Yoda to our own life and a Jedi to everyone else's. But how do we become more mindful?

Mindfulness can be broken into six core aspects:

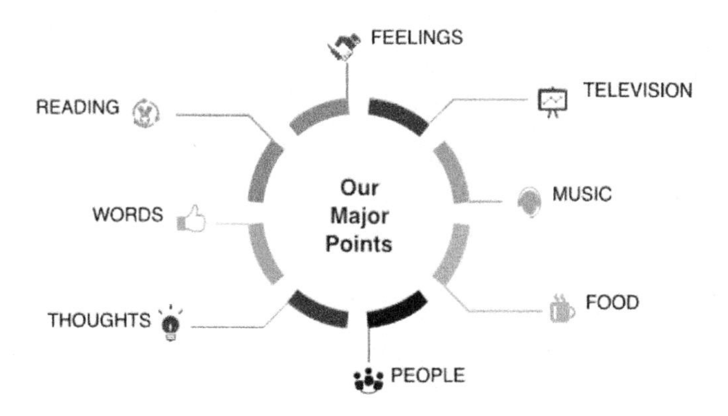

## Thoughts

It is believed by many experts that humans have about 50,000–70,000 thoughts per day, and as many as 98 percent of those thoughts are exactly the same as the day before. That's a lot of repetition happening.

So, the real question is: What is the *quality* of your thoughts? Are you typically thinking positive, productive, uplifting thoughts? Or, are they negative and worrisome? Unfortunately, most of us are consumed with the latter. Negative thoughts become habit that we don't even realize we have until we are challenged with becoming more mindful of our inner dialogue.

I have found that many cases of depression or chronic sadness come from this type of negative rumination. It's an addictive thought cycle that keeps playing over and over. This negative thought cycle becomes truth, even when it is not truthful. But the good news is that can happen on the opposite end of the spectrum with positive, productive thoughts, too. We just have to make a conscious choice to become more aware of what we are primarily thinking and consciously commit to changing what we want to improve.

**Our thoughts are anchored in our beliefs, so beginning to recognize our thoughts can give us greater insights to our beliefs.**

As I mentioned in the last chapter, beliefs begin to be projected on us when we are born by those around us. Many of those beliefs become programmed deeply in our subconscious minds. We are unaware of many beliefs that run our lives because they are so deep in our subconscious mind and have been a part of who we are for so long. It becomes just how we live and view the world. Tying this together, it's helpful to understand that our beliefs create our perceptions, and our perceptions become our thoughts. These thoughts become our "reality" until we realize:

**Our perceptions are not the truth, just interpretations from the past that create assumptions in our present.**

(I will get into this more in later chapters.) The really important thing I want you to understand here is that we consistently need to audit our beliefs around things to change our thoughts and change our realities. If you catch yourself thinking thought patterns you would like to change, evaluate what your beliefs are around that thought pattern, so you can change the belief and change the thought pattern.

A great way to create thought pattern disruption is to practice the **Mental Reset Button** technique.

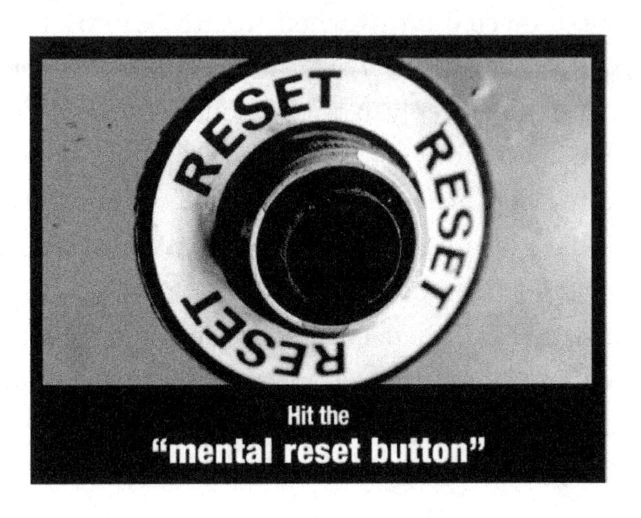


When you catch yourself in a thought process that you know is not supportive of your desires, instantly visualize a delete button and imagine yourself pressing the delete button three times. You can actually say, "Delete!" out loud three times as well. Then replace the negative thought with a more positive, productive thought. As you begin this process, have two or three pre-prepared thoughts you can switch to. I call these **Back-Pocket Thoughts**. For example, if you find yourself saying something like, "What if I fail?" instantly replace it with, "What if I succeed?" and then begin to visualize how that positive experience could look.

When my daughters were 5, they were riding around the house on their new scooters. My one daughter Morgan kept falling. With frustration, she looked at me and said, "Mom, I am having a really bad day!" I replied excitedly with an opportunity to teach a big life lesson. "Well Morgan, if you believe that and keep saying that, what do you think will keep happening?" She asked with a question in her voice, "I will get more of a bad day?" I said, "That's right! You need to hit the mental reset button and delete your negative thoughts and re-program with something more positive to turn your day around like, "I only have good days!" As I told her to delete her negative thoughts, I kept making a tapping motion on my forehead while saying "delete" to give her more visual clues to make it a more concrete lesson. She looked at me with determination and began to tap her head saying "Delete," then continued walking around repeating, "I only have good days!"

She picked up her scooter with her new perspective, and wouldn't you know, a few minutes later her twin sister ran over her foot with her scooter. She stopped and with a frustrated shout said, "Madison, I only have good days!" She then came over to me and asked, "Mom, if I said 'I only have good days,' then why did Madison run over my foot?" Holding back my giggles from the cuteness of this all, I knew I had a great opportunity to drive this lesson home. I said, "Well Morgan, I don't believe you really believed it, and you have to believe it first and more importantly, you gave your power away to her, when the power is in your control. You get to see it how YOU want to see it. It's called your perspective. We always get to choose how we want to see something. That's one of our special powers that most people give away to others!"

The only thing we really have control of in life is our perspectives, which are directly tied to our thoughts. If the rumination of most of our thoughts are negative or worrisome, it is because that's how we are choosing to view our world. The fastest way to take control of your thoughts is to choose to master your ability to more positive and productive perspectives to everything going on around you. This can instantly flip the "victim mentality" into being healthier and happier. Once we improve our thoughts, we improve how we feel, we improve our reality. The more and more we get better at this, even not-so-good situations can be made better by how we chose to see them.

Another way to help train our brains to stay in more productive thought processes is to practice gratitude daily. Not only is this good for our brain training by creating new neural pathways in the brain, but it increases the neurotransmitter dopamine which makes us feels good, therefore almost instantly enhancing our emotional and physical state.

Gratitude requires appreciation of the positive aspects of your life. The more we consciously commit to doing this, the more it becomes innate over time. We can train our brains to view the world through an improved lens. This, in turn, makes life a heck of a lot more enjoyable.

Many years ago, I read a book called *Power vs. Force* by David Hawkins, MD, Ph D. In the book, Hawkins quantifies the energy of various emotional states. Love is the highest, with appreciation being right under love and gratitude being right under appreciation. I found it to be so interesting that appreciation has a greater energy frequency than gratitude, because I realized that appreciation is the active expression of gratitude. Acknowledging that love has the highest frequency, the real question for me became, "How do I get closest to the frequency of love from the place of gratitude more often?"

So I created what I call the **I LOVE Exercise.** Like any new activity, I encourage you to make this a habit. The best way to quickly make something a habit is through frequency and consistency, so I suggest you set an alarm a few times a day to do this—it only takes two minutes.

To begin, identify something you want to focus on. (Eventually you will be able to focus on anything at all and successfully do the exercise.) Once you choose your focus, you will begin going down an emotionally evoking journey, which is different than just writing down something you are grateful for. Here is an example:

If I just wrote down in my gratitude journal, "I am grateful for my kids," it may raise my frequency a little, but only for a brief moment because I didn't connect to why I am grateful for them or all the things I am grateful for about them.

Instead I begin with, "I LOVE my children. I love hearing their belly laughter coming from their bedrooms. I love hearing them have conversations with each other and helping each other out. I love that whoever is ready first in the morning helps the one who isn't by getting their breakfast and snacks for the day. I love when we all lay on the couch together and watch a movie like when they were little, and I love that I feel connected and close in their teen world." I could go on and on, but do you see how I am identifying visual memories and images that are emotionally evoking? This method raises my energy frequency so much higher.

One other example I like to use is the beach—because I really love the beach! I love being on the beach first thing in the morning when the sun is rising and the sun's warmth is hitting my face. I love that the sand is smooth and there are barely any footprints in it yet. I love walking along the water and hearing the ocean. I love putting my chair in the sand right along the shore line and watching the water go in and out. I love listening to families arrive on the beach ready to make new memories. I love watching the excitement in kids' faces when they arrive at the beach. I love when the sun is ready to set on the beach as the evening air feels cooler. Here, you can see the visual journey of my emotional connection to the beach. You can feel all of the many layers of the beach. By doing this exercise, I can essentially go to the beach, both emotionally and physiologically, without actually having gone to the beach. It helps me reframe my thoughts when negative emotions and impulses try to take control. Open up your journal and do a few I LOVE exercises. Make this a daily habit. Life becomes so much more pleasurable when you do this each day.

Another strategy that can be helpful when learning how to be more in control of our thoughts is making notes. A lot of people say that many of their thoughts are consumed with future-tripping, which means they are consumed with all of the things they need to do next. I battle this by making notes. The second something comes to mind, let it go by writing it down in a notebook. If you don't have a notebook available, text it to yourself.

If you desire to get MORE everything good in life, it begins with the quality of thoughts that you are thinking!

## Words

Words put our thoughts into motion, giving them even more energy. I tell my children all the time, "Do not think about what you don't want, think about what you **do** want. And certainly do not speak about what you don't want, only breathe into life what you **do** want."

This is a fundamental principle of quantum physics called the Law of Attraction. To demystify this for any naysayers, I would like to clarify that the Law of Attraction is how I am writing this book. The Law of Attraction is how I have accomplished pretty much everything I have done, especially the big things.

I was blessed to encounter a man named Bob Proctor back in 2000, who was speaking at a conference I was attending. EVERY word he said resonated with me so deeply, I had to meet him and learn more about what he had to say. After he was done speaking, I fought my way through the crowd to meet him and tell him I needed to learn more from him. He instructed me to connect with his assistant that Monday morning and find out how to learn more. His assistant then told me about a mastermind group called "The 3% Club" that Bob and Mark Victor Hansen were starting the following week in LA. I really had no business (logically) dropping everything at the last minute, investing in mastermind program, and taking off to LA after just getting back from a work trip in Canada, but thank goodness I did! The program and all of its teachings upleveled my life in ways I could never have imagined. I share many of those teachings with you today in my own iteration. One of the biggest lessons I learned was this: **do not focus on what you don't want, only what you do want.**

The words we use are powerful in what we create. They are also great insight to the psychological state we are at. When I invite someone to an event and they say, "I will try to make it," I immediately cross them off the list because their words told me that they weren't committed to coming.

If I were to tell you, "I am going to lose 15 pounds this year!" and someone else told you, "I will try to lose 15 pounds this year," which person would you have more faith in? Of course you will believe the person who says, "I will." They are breathing life into their goal.

If you desire to increase your mindfulness to get MORE of everything you desire in life, the words you choose matter. As you are becoming more mindful of the quality of the words you are choosing you might want to find someone in your life who you know is already mindful and ask them to hold you accountable and call you out of they hear you using low quality language. Or you can take an class on Neuro-Linguistic Programming to help you become more aware.

## Feelings

How many times has someone asked you how you are feeling and you pull for a short list of answers? Or how many times have you asked others how they are feeling and they pulled from a similar short list of answers?

So many people in our society are out of touch with their emotional states. Please know, I do not mean to be rude in making this statement. I simply hope to wake people up about how important emotional awareness actually is.

The sad fact is that many of us were told NOT to feel in our childhood. Boys are told not to cry. Women are scolded in the workplace for being "too emotional" and it is the status quo to be numb. This phenomenon is turning us into walking zombies — numbing to escape our emotional range because we are simply unaware of how to process it all. That is certainly not a world I want to live in, which is why I advocate for social and emotional intelligence education in school, starting in pre-school. The world would be such a better place.

How many human emotions do you believe exist? If you said six, you are not alone, as that what was previously believed. But we are way more emotionally complex.

According to a study from the Greater Good Science, faculty director Dachner Keltner suggests that there are actually at least 27 distinct emotions—which are all intimately interconnected with each other. (cited www.greatergood.berkley.edu) Emotional experiences are extremely layered and complex and integrate so many meanings from our past and present—all while being affected by our current physiological state. Often, what we are upset about in the current moment is actually attached to unresolved issues from our past. Our emotions are impacted by how we feel. For example, if we are hungry or exhausted it will amplify the situation. Becoming more mindful of our emotions and our physiological state and how it affects our emotions or the meaning we are assigning to our emotions is one of the most powerful ways to navigate and control how we feel.

To become more masterful at controlling our emotions, we must first be able to pause to identify them, assess why we are feeling what we are feeling, then choose what new meaning (if any) we would like to assign.

## checklist

**Why do I feel this way?**
(emotional awareness)

**Is it real? Or my ego running the show?**
(ego awareness)

**Where is it coming from?**
(trigger awareness)

**How could I see it differently?**
(shift in perspective)

**What am I supposed to be learning?**
(wisdom)

Here is a list of some normal emotions and behaviors. On the left side are the more emotionally unintelligent ones and one the right side is the inversion or opposite feelings/behaviors. When trying to great better patterns you can look at this chart and try to figure out a better pattern.

| EUI | EI |
|---|---|
| Expectations | Acceptance |
| Judgment | Inspiration |
| Fear | Freedom |
| Blame | Perspective Shift |
| Withdraw | Engage Intimacy |
| Attack | Heal |
| Anger | Forgiveness |
| Complacency | Appreciation |
| Entitlement | Gratitude |
| Defensiveness | Openness |
| Manipulation | Faith |
| Isolation | Immersion |
| Unhappiness | Happy |
| Emptiness | Peace |
| Intolerance | Compassion |
| Insensitivity | Empathy |

**It is also important to acknowledge that different people have varying capacities for each emotion.**

This can be challenging for many of us to understand and respect because it is hard to grasp how someone isn't as loving as us, or as thoughtful as we are, or as patient. But the truth is that someone else's 100 percent capacity of patience may only be your 20 percent.

My father was born into an emotionally unavailable family. He continued that cycle and was an emotionally unavailable father (although he improved in his advanced age). However, when I was younger, I was angry that my father wasn't as affectionate and adoring as my friends' dads were. I felt slighted and disappointed constantly because I compared him to other fathers and created expectations that he should be the same. Once I realized that the expectations I placed on my dad were what was causing me the most pain, I changed them and was able to see things a lot differently. I realized that my dad was loving me at his 100 percent capacity and I was able to gain a greater understanding that he was doing his best. That understanding helped me shift my emotions from anger and disappointment to compassion and empathy.

Emotional capacity can change. It is not something that is fixed forever, as I mentioned my dad became way more emotionally available in his older age, but his capacity had to expand over time, experiences, and desire.

The more mindful and effective we become with identifying and processing our emotions and their capacities, the more we can be in **emotional harmony**. This is how resiliency is created.

Resiliency is such an important emotional skill set to develop for emotional regulation. Processing skills are so incredibly important, yet most people lack them. I find that the people who are most skilled at processing their emotions are those who have overcome a lot of adversity and continued to rise above it. Those who struggle the most are those who choose to fall victim to their circumstances and blame others. And then there are people who just don't know what they don't know, and just need some processing tools put into their toolbox and will thrive to the highest levels. This book is a tool for you to build the best version of **self.**

A side note: For those of you who are parents, becoming better at identifying and expressing your emotions isn't just good for you, but is a great thing to model for your children early on so that they can learn how to assess and process their emotions early on.

The more we are aware of our emotional state and manage our emotions, not only are we healthier and happier, our relationships are more harmonious and we get more out of life every day.

To get MORE of everything good you desire, you must become more mindful of how you feel and how that affects what you do.

## Foods and Overall Nutrition

What you eat and drink affects how you feel. How much you eat and drink affects how you feel. Every time you put something into your body, you create a chemical reaction that can change your moods and energy levels. Many of us never make the connection between what or how much we are eating and our personalities and performance, therefore unknowingly minimizing our performance in life. In becoming more mindful of our nutrition, we have more power and control over our lives and our outcomes to get MORE of everything good.

We will discuss this in more depth in the next chapter.

## People

One of the best lessons I learned from my mentor, T. Harv Eker, was, "Your network is your net worth—physically, financially, mentally, emotionally, and spiritually."

Your **"default-self"** is the sum of the people and experiences that influenced your childhood.

A vast majority of our programming happened in the first 7 years of our lives. We were programmed by the people who were around us, as well as the things we were watching on television and reading about.

This is where many of our beliefs began, whether we agreed with them or not, they became our truths—**our paradigms**. As we become mindful adults, we become aware of many of these programmed beliefs and behaviors that do not serve us.

When we desire to change those beliefs and behaviors, we must surround ourselves with people who hold the beliefs and values we desire to become. We need to be surrounded by people who challenge our limited beliefs, who expose us to more expansive beliefs, and who expose us to ways of life that we desire for ourselves. We must surround ourself with people who can lovingly call us out when our less than optimal selves show up. People who lift us up, not drag us down.

In short: **detox the drainers and increase the enhancers.** Our default-self will still show up in moments when we are triggered, full of fear, or are just plain ignorant to a behavior that is comfortable to us. But the more we surround ourselves with people who already are what we aspire to be, we can see when our default-self and can allow a "new" self to show up more clearly. We will also expand our world view and what is possible by surrounding ourselves with the people who are already living more expansively.

The opposite of expansive relationships are the ones that derail our efforts with toxic drama. I choose to live in the **drama-free zone,**

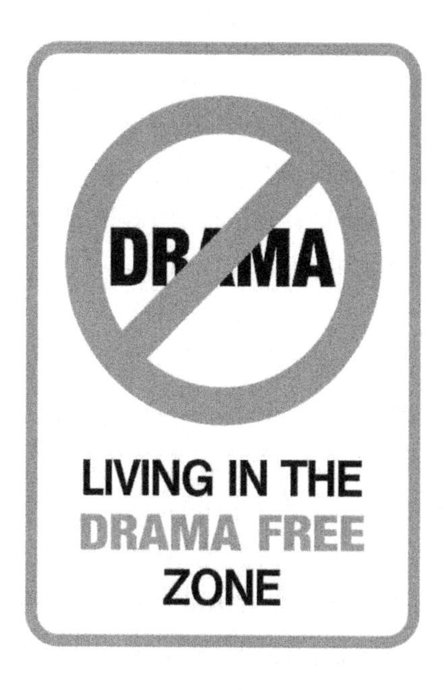


and anyone who knows me knows how serious I am about that. And guess what? It actually helps others around me to rise to be the best version of who they are if there is no drama. It also quickly eliminates the people who drain your energy, happiness, and productivity.

I have programmed my daughters with this same belief system since they were toddlers. Now, as teenagers, they clearly identify and steer clear of people and circumstances that create drama (as much as possible for teenagers). When I ask why they don't hang out with certain people, they will often respond, "They cause too much drama, Mom!" and BAM! I know it worked.

I know many of you are thinking, "Okay Jen, I want to live in the drama-free zone, and I want to only surround myself with people who help me become the best version of myself. But what about the family, friends, and co-workers I can't break free from?"

For the people who you are unable to remove from your life for whatever reason, you must change your **expectations** of them in order to be free of disappointments and disruption to your evolutions.

**The biggest lesson here is that our expectations of others is the number one thing to cause self-inflicted pain in our lives.**

As I mentioned earlier, my dad had limited emotional capacity around being affectionate, so if I expected him to behave affectionately, I would be disappointed and hurt. But that would be my own self-inflicted pain based on my expectations of how someone should behave. For a long time, I was hurt by this—until I realized **I am responsible for my**

**expectations and how they make me feel. People cannot think like us, act like us, or be how we expect them to be; they are how they are.** Just as someone else's emotional capacity can differ from our own, how someone behaves based on their life experiences can vastly differ from how you expect them to behave, so adjusting expectations is key to our own happiness.

In order to get MORE of everything good in life, we need to let go of the expectations of others to think like us, act like us, respond like us, or worse...live to please us and make us happy.

We will discuss expectations more deeply in Chapter 5.

## Free time

Just as who you spend your time with is important to your personal growth and evolution, so is how you spend your free time.

Do you waste hours of your life watching mindless television? Or hours of your life worrying about what everyone else is doing? Or just plain wasting time?

I have a huge secret to share with all of you. You ready for it? This is a game changer for so many:

**Growth equals happiness.**

**Let me say it again so that you can really process it: Growth equals happiness.**

So many of us waste time doing mindless, unproductive things thinking that it will make us happy. Instead, we find ourselves bored, stuck, disconnected, and unfulfilled. The reality is that happiness comes from our own personal growth; for example, learning new things, seeing new perspectives, accomplishing new skills, and producing results.

So why then do so many avoid doing things that actually bring these results. Many subconsciously see growth as "work," instead of something exciting that should be cherished. I believe a lot of these beliefs systems begin by:

- Watching our parents and/or community living this way
- Being influenced early in life that "school isn't fun!", and therefore learning isn't fun.
- A universal portrayal that you can either "work" or "play", but you can't have both at the same time.

- Thinking that "having fun" is synonymous with wasting time doing mindless things—

often things that numb our senses as a form of escape

If children learn early on that growth is what creates happiness, our world would look very different. We wouldn't need to do so many things to escape our reality, because our reality would be so much more fulfilling and rewarding. For example, I chose the life of an entrepreneur because I watched so many adults who were unhappy in their lives, checking in and out of life daily like robots. People lived for Fridays and cried on Mondays. But I refused to buy into the belief that life is supposed to be a mediocre journey of existing to pay bills. I refused to buy into the belief that life is supposed to be one long hardship full of pain and suffering. I refused to believe I was supposed to just do what I got my degree in and live in a box society ignorantly created. As a young adult I knew that that was not the existence I wanted, and I believed I could choose to do something that made me happy every day. So I did. I chose to believe I could create my happiness by doing things I loved, and then even the hard days brought joy and fulfillment through accomplishment. I believed I could continue learning and taking on challenges every day to keep sculpting the life I desired. I spent my free time, learning, exploring, meeting new people, seeing new things and living. Every day hasn't been easy but it sure has been fulfilling. I know for sure that this lifestyle works. It is the only way to design the ultimate forms of success. Not just financial success, but more importantly, lives of consistent happiness, fulfillment and inner peace.

In order to get MORE of everything good out of life, we need to be aware and intentional of how we spend our free time. We must make more conscious choices to do things that fuel our souls and make us feel alive every day!

## The Power of Mindfulness

**Mindfulness is the foundation to intentional living.**

It's the awareness and strength to make more conscious choices. It's the understanding that many aspects of life are in our control, and we can exercise that power daily! Mindfulness allows us to identify and remove the things that blocks us from what we desire. It is the gateway to helping us master our mindsets.

**When we master our mindset, we master our lives.**

Make mindful living your biggest commitment today, and everything else will begin to fall into place.

**This isn't a path of perfection, but a more conscious way of living, so when we do "mess up," we can *course-correct* faster.**

## Journaling Prompts

1) What storms have you encountered that challenged you to rise stronger and more powerful? What impact has it had on your life today?

2) List at least three "back-pocket thoughts" which can help you transform negative thoughts into positive, productive thoughts. What negative thoughts do you frequently have that will require using the "mental reset button"?

3) Practice the "I LOVE Exercise" with at least three things you are grateful for. How did this exercise help you gain a deeper appreciation for those things?

4) As I said earlier, words put our thoughts into motion. Put into words a list of the deepest desires you have today.

5) Check out the list of 27 human emotions. For each emotion on the list, identify a situation in which you felt that emotion.

6) Catalogue every item you eat and drink for one day. How do you think those foods impacted

your personality and performance throughout the day?

7) Who are the five people you surround yourself with the most often? Do they reflect the life you desire? If you could choose, who would you ideally place in those five slots? How can you make that happen?

8) How do you typically spend your free time? How can you transform that time to be more stimulating for your learning and growth while still getting the rest you need?

CHAPTER 4

# OPTIMIZATION

## of Body & Brain

We have all heard the saying, "Your body is a temple," but most never truly embody the values of what that means. I do not mean this from a religious perspective, but from the perspective of self-love. A temple, by definition, is "a place dedicated to worship." By definition, worship means, "a feeling or expression of reverence and adoration." And the definition of reverence is, "deep respect for someone or something." So I ask you this: do you treat your body like a temple? Do you have reverence for the value of your body and what it does for you on a daily basis? I am not saying you have to be "perfect" every day. **Again, this isn't about a path of perfection, but rather a path of greater consciousness: making more conscious choices on a daily basis that nourish your body and mind, which in turn will optimize who you are and what you are capable of every day.**

The one area we have the most control over in our lives is how we treat our bodies. Often when people are young, they feel invincible. Our bodies are more resilient and can handle more "abusive" behavior. Unfortunately, it's not until most people get older (if ever) that they realize they aren't invincible and wish they had taken better care of their bodies from early on.

More and more cultures, especially the American culture, abuse their bodies with a litany of toxic, chemical-filled, high-sugar foods, drinks, and other substances on a daily basis. Many are also highly sleep-deprived and dehydrated. They keep challenging their systems, expecting their bodies to just keep supporting them... until it doesn't. People feel entitled to their bodies' power instead of appreciative and respectful of its miracles. Many think that feeling chronically tired is "just the way it is." Many are chronically ill, also assuming that's "just life", not realizing it doesn't have to be that way. They never realize that simply eating and living a lifestyle that supports one's immune system not only makes one healthier but also happier, more energized, more mentally clear, more focused, and therefore able to be more productive and enjoy life a lot MORE. The sad thing is that so many people don't even know how good it feels to feel good on a regular basis, because they have lived in a mediocre state of energy and well-being for so long.

Without our health we have nothing. I know this firsthand because, when I was 25 years of age, my body was challenged in a way many don't experience until they are a lot older. As I mentioned in Chapter 1, my first career path was in the fitness industry. I was obsessed with exercise, to the point that I over-exercised. At that time, I was teaching about 3 high impact aerobics classes every day, about 5 days a week. And that's not to mention lifting, working out alongside my clients, and doing regular yoga classes to stay flexible. Quite honestly, I thought I was invincible. My business colleagues and clients would call me "Super Groover", and I spent every day trying to live up to that name. I was chronically over-training and overworking. But the people around me reinforced that behavior by encouraging it, is if it was something to be proud of.

At 45 years of age, I can look back and see how stupid I was.

In early 2000 I trained for two back-to-back competitions: the National Aerobic Championship and the Galaxy Fitness Competition. They were two very different types of competitions. One demanded more aerobic training while the other called for more anaerobic training. Two different energy systems. Two totally different types of training. Yet, I did both. So silly. Most fitness competitors will feel a brief period of exhaustion after competitions are over—both mental and physical. However, after the two competitions were over, my exhaustion stayed and stayed. No matter what I did, no matter how much I slept, I felt exhausted, mentally foggy, and somewhat depressed. I was severely lacking any sense of motivation and struggled to feel passionate about anything—neither was a normal experience for my personality. Long story short, after a long scavenger hunt of trying to figure out what was wrong with me, many doctors threw their hands up as to why I was feeling the way I was. Many told me it was in my head, confused as to how I would look like such an essence of health on the outside—all while I felt like I was dying a slow death on the inside. I eventually learned that I had developed several autoimmune suppression issues. One of these was Hashimoto's Disease, which can be a serious autoimmune disease of the thyroid which causes many issues, including chronic exhaustion, memory loss, moodiness, and hair loss, just to name a few things. During the height of this health crisis, I learned something that many don't realize until later in life when it's too late:

**Your health is the foundation of everything else. Without it, your work, relationships, and quality of life ALL suffer.**

This realization was a such a gift because it made me understand the significant value of what I am teaching you today: nothing feels as good as good energy feels. Life is much sweeter and more fulfilling when we are healthy. The healthier we are, the more we enjoy every aspect of life. So when I suggest eating healthier, staying hydrated, or creating better patterns for quality sleep, don't think I'm trying to "take your fun away." I hope you realize these actions will actually be adding way more fun to your life.

Eventually I reversed the damage I'd caused by living a lifestyle that supported the strength of my immune system. At 45, I have way more energy and vitality than I ever did in my 20's and early 30's.

During that time period, I feverishly read everything I could get my hands on about autoimmune issues. I asked as many health practitioners as possible for their insights. One particular book I read significantly changed my life: *Heal Yourself, Heal Your Life* by Louise Hay.

What I started to realize after reading the book was that, while I looked like the essence of health on the outside, it was an illusion masking the reality. My "fitness" lifestyle wasn't really wellness. It was more like self-abuse. This ongoing beating up on my body (masked as exercise) in addition to my never-ending strive for perfection was really a form of control and abuse that was masked as something positive. My unhealed childhood trauma was still affecting my physical, mental, and emotional states. But on the outside, it all seemed healthy, so not only was it acceptable, but it was continuously reinforced by positive affirmations and compliments from others. It was no different than the physiological abuse one creates by emotionally eating to the point of obesity, aside from the fact that my struggle was disguised as fitness. The truth is, being truly fit is about being healthy and well: mentally, physically and emotionally. Today, I prefer the term "wellness" versus "fitness" because I believe, for many, they create two different underlying connotations. One aims for overall wellbeing; the other aims at external vanity.

Truly taking charge of our power to get MORE of everything we desire in life begins with **simple self-love, self-respect, and appreciation of what are bodies and minds are capable of when fueled and supported properly.**

**When we optimize our physiological state, we instantly optimize our mental and emotional states.**

Do you ever feel upset about something and indulge in a big bowl of ice cream to "feel better'? One may feel a momentary pleasure from the sugar surge, but ultimately, once our blood sugar begins to drop, we actually feel worse. This worsens our emotional state and perhaps our mental state, especially if one begins beating themselves up over the large calorie indulgence.

Ever go out to lunch in the middle of the work day and eat a high-carb meal with things like breads or pasta? Once you came back to the office, did you notice how you were feeling? Most likely exhausted, irritable, and less productive. The sad thing is that most people never make the connection that what they ate at lunch is sabotaging their well-intentioned efforts for a productive afternoon. Even worse, as the lull sets in, they seek a sugary substance for a short term "boost", not realizing that they have yet again exacerbated their energy roller coaster, making it harder to sustain energy, focus, and be productive. Once again, they are living with the belief that "this is a normal afternoon energy slump" and not realizing that their choices created it. In my latest TEDx Talk, I share the story of what helped me break a life-long sugar addiction by understanding the mindset above. This talk can be viewed from the link on my website jengroover.com. As we become more conscious of how the food we eat makes us feel, along with the correct portion sizes for our bodies' sizes, we can make better choices to fuel our bodies and brains in a more productive way. We shift the addiction from the sugar highs to something more useful—becoming addicted to feeling good, enjoying life more with high energy, mental clarity and hyper-focus.

I personally prefer to go through life working smarter instead of harder, so I make more conscious choices, especially when I need to be productive. I optimize my physiological state with what I put in my mouth, how I sleep, staying active, hydrating, oxygenating, detoxifying, and supporting my immune system. Below is an image you can keep in a visible spot as a reminder, so that you, too, can work smarter instead of harder to get MORE of everything you desire in life.

Just like I created an auditing system for becoming more Mindful, I have created an auditing system for you to improve your physiological state, which will in turn improve your mental and emotional states.

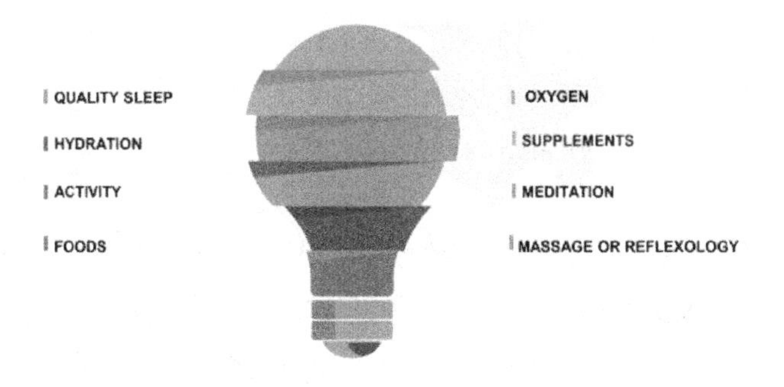


Remember, there are very few things in the world that we have control over, but how we treat our body is one thing we can control.

## Nutrition

First thing on this list is nutrition, because this is one thing people seem to struggle with the most. Every time we eat or drink something, we cause a chemical reaction in our body. Most don't think of it that way, but it's something to become really aware of. Are most of the chemical reactions you are causing hurting you or helping you?

Your brain is always "on." It works hard around the clock, even while you're asleep. This means your brain requires a constant supply of fuel. That "fuel" comes from the foods you eat — and what's in that fuel makes all the difference. What you eat directly affects the structure and function of your brain and your mood.

Your brain functions best when it gets the best kind of fuel. Eating high-quality foods that contain lots of vitamins, minerals, and antioxidants nourishes the brain and protects it from oxidative stress — the "waste" (free radicals) produced when the body uses oxygen, which can damage cells.

Unfortunately, your brain can be damaged by choosing anything other than this good fuel. The substances produced from lower grade fuels, like processed or refined foods, cause the brain to malfunction. Diets high in refined sugars promote inflammation and oxidative stress. Multiple studies have found a correlation between a diet high in refined sugars and impaired brain function — and even a worsening of symptoms of mood disorders, such as depression.

Today, the field of nutritional psychiatry is finding there are many consequences and correlations between what you eat, how you feel, and how you behave.

## Activity

Staying active is an important part of optimizing your physiological state. This isn't a lesson on becoming the leanest, most fit person in the room, but a lesson on connecting the dots to how your activity level is hurting you or helping you. Remember, our goal here is to recognize how our daily lifestyle habits can enhance (or diminish) our energy, mental clarity, and ability to perform at higher levels consistently to maximize our potential and simply enjoy life MORE.

Staying active doesn't mean you have to beat yourself up at the gym. It could simply mean walking every day and doing some weight bearing exercises, both of which can be incorporated into your day (which removes the "I am too busy" excuses).

While I do enjoy going to fitness classes, my schedule is often too complex to allow for classes. When that happens, I plan my activity into my work day. I often to walk meetings or make phone calls while I am walking. I can add in some squats and lunges at my desk. Or, if I am working from home, I can add in some step runs, pushups, and sit ups to break up each task. A workout doesn't need to be done all at once. Have some fun with it. Let it break up your to-do list if need be. If you hate the workouts you have carved out for yourself, you will most likely procrastinate doing them. The key is to get moving, get your blood flowing, get your heart rate elevated, uptake the oxygen levels to your lungs and brain, and get some adrenaline going. If you feel a midday slump, go for a walk or do some jumping jacks. I assure you, you will get revved back up quickly to optimize your afternoon and evening. Of course, these are general suggestions that each individual may have to consult with their physician on.

## Sleep

Consistent, high-quality sleep helps our bodies and brains recover each night so that we can optimize our performance the next day. We all know how cranky and mentally unclear we can feel after a poor night of sleep, or multiple nights of poor sleep. Our bodies and brains work so much harder just to function on those days, and it certainly prohibits us from optimizing who we are and getting MORE of everything we desire in life, especially if it is a chronic issue. As a culture that burns the candle at both ends, it seems much of our society suffers from sleep deprivation. While it might seem "normal", it is hazardous to your health both short and long term.

According to the Harvard Medical School, Sleep Medicine Division, "Short term lack of sleep can affect judgement, mood, ability to learn and retain information and may increase serious risk of accidents and injury. In the long term, chronic sleep deprivation may lead to a host of health problems including obesity, diabetes, cardiovascular disease, and even early mortality," (www.healthysleep.med. harvard.edu). With all of this information, why on earth would we knowingly not prioritize our sleep?

This falls in line with my firm belief in creating a habit to consistently "work smarter, then harder." When we value this habit, we can truly optimize our mental clarity and be more productive.

I know many people have a lot of issues around sleep for various reasons, so I am going to address some of the most common ones to try to solve some problems for anyone who struggles to get a consistent good night's sleep.

1) **Routine:** Creating a consistent bedtime routine is one of the best ways to get good sleep. Ever hear of Pavlov's Dog? Well, we are the same when we create routines. Our

bodies can anticipate what is going to happen next. This is a simple adjustment that many never even think about incorporating into their lives. Think of every baby book that gives advice on getting your baby to sleep through the night—the top thing every expert suggests is creating a bedtime routine. Adults, while we are older, still thrive in the sleep arena with a routine.

As a great example, if you want to be asleep by 10:30, begin your routine at 10:00. Go upstairs, wash up with dimmed lights (sight senses), maybe have a scent you spray (olfactory senses), perhaps put on some lavender lotion (touch senses) and listen to a meditation (auditory senses) or turn on a box fan (I will come back to that in a moment). The more you get your senses involved the more the body will feel the "cues" happening and anticipate the sleep that is coming next.

2) **White Noise:** White noise is helpful to get a deeper rest. The white noise blocks out sounds that could suddenly wake us up. Babies sleep better with white noise because

it creates a womb-like sound. Why wouldn't the same be for adults? I personally use a good, old-fashioned box fan that creates a louder, more "solid" white noise than sound machines ever could.

3) **Lavender:** I mentioned lavender lotion, but it's not just the lotion that lulls you to sleep. Research has proven that lavender helps people get into a deeper sleep. I use a toxic-free lavender spray on my pillow. You can use lavender oil on your body or in a bath before bed, or have a lavender candle lit while you do your bedtime routine.

4) **Technology:** A key factor in regulating your body's natural biorhythms has to do with light. Too much light before bed can keep you from feeling tired or getting a restful night's sleep. It is extremely helpful to stop looking at your phone before bed and turn off the tv and lights. I know some people think they need the TV on to sleep, but it is proven that this causes disruptive sleep from a sound and light (blue light) perspective. Once I learned this, I removed the TV in my room so that I wouldn't even be tempted to

watch. Also, try to keep your phone away from your bed. There are many reasons to do this for your well-being.

## Hydration

We are a chronically dehydrated society. Most people do not drink enough water. Yes, I said water; not coffee, tea, soda, juices—but water. Since our bodies are mostly compromised of water, our bodies have to work harder to sustain normal functioning when we are dehydrated. It's actually critical to our heart health. Keeping the body hydrated helps our blood to pump through the blood vessels to our muscles more effortlessly. Not only does dehydration make our hearts work harder; it makes our brains work harder. Often when people have headaches or can't think clearly, it's a sign of dehydration. They just need to drink some water to feel better.

If you are thirsty, you are already dehydrated. What each person needs to stay hydrated varies based on body weight, climate, activity levels, how many caffeinated or alcoholic drinks you may have had, etc. A good practice is to stay aware of the color of your urine; pale is good, darker color means you need to drink more water.

The more you stay hydrated, the better your body and brain work, and the MORE you can get out of life.

## Oxygen

Cognitive improvements have been recorded in patients who use at home oxygen therapy. However. these findings can also be linked to research that suggests exercise will make you smarter because it increases the amount of oxygen travelling to your brain (oxygenworldwide.com). We don't need to have an oxygen machine at home to make use of this valuable information; we just need to become more intentional breathers.

A new saying in the medical world is, "Sitting is the new smoking," because as we sit, we often hunch over and begin to take shallow breaths. Over time, this can cause a serious lack of good oxygen flow. This can eventually become chronic oxygen deprivation, which can create toxic buildup in our bodies. Getting quality and a good quantity of oxygen to our brains can be one of the fastest ways to become "smarter." Can you guess the fastest way to do this? Force a yawn! Yes, that's right, when we force a yawn, we can create a great uptake of oxygen to our brains, instantly helping us work smarter rather than harder. I have implemented this bio-hack in my life and use this technique before speaking, pitch meetings, important phone calls, etc. If you want to be more productive, I suggest adding it into your life too.

## Supplements

I could write on the importance of this topic forever because there are so many types of supplements and so many nutrient deficiencies in our society, but I am going to keep it simple.

No matter how well you eat, to get proper nutrition these days, we need to supplement our diets. There are tests that you can get done to analyze what nutrients you are deficient in. This is the ideal way to proceed, but if you choose not to do this, do make sure to take high-quality, highly soluble (digestible) daily supplements. Yes, this will cost you a little more money, but it is worth it for your health. This will prevent health problems before they happen. I often laugh because so many people scowl at paying extra for quality supplements and choose the cheap stuff (which is a TOTAL waste of money), but won't think twice about dropping the same amount of money on crappy food or alcohol. Remember, when we are nutrient deficient, our bodies work way harder rather than smarter to thrive and get more out of life.

## Meditation

For many years, I would listen to people talk about the importance of meditation and watch people in mediation classes seemingly so connected with their inner-zen. I would be in awe—and quite jealous. I would think, "Are they really not thinking? Is there really silence in their heads right now?"

You do not need to go far to find the incredible amount of evidence that proves the importance of mediation in our daily lives. Learning about this research created a great sense of value and desire for me to make it part of my daily routine, but it was a lot harder for me than it seemed for so many others. I felt like I was wasting time because I never quite felt I was "doing it right." But then I was turned onto Binaural Beats as a way of meditating and it was amazing. Binaural Beats can quickly change the brains state. It is often referred to as sound wave therapy. It makes use of the fact that the right and left each hear a slightly different frequency tone, yet the brain perceives it as one sound. There are various binaural beats to choose from depending on the results you are looking for; from deeper sleep to calming/restorative, to increase concentration, increase energy and decrease anxiety and more. I have found binaural beats as a "meditative' exercise that is incredibly helpful for me.

I believe in the benefits of mediation. I used to think, "I don't have time for that! Who has time just to sit still and do nothing!" until I learned we really are doing "something" when we meditate. We are rejuvenating our brains and for all of you over-achievers this helps you do more, faster. The way I started to envision it was, think of your brain like a closet. In the morning when you wake up after a good night's sleep your brain is like a clean and organized closet. By the middle of a busy day, our brains are more like a messy closet with clothes and shoes thrown everywhere. When we go into the clean closet, it's easy to find things (like the files in our brains) but by the middle of the day it gets harder to access the files because our brains are more like the messy, cluttered closet after being bombarded with information all day. If we "clean up the closet" though, the rest of the day is easier and more productive because it's easier to access the resources of our brains. For me, mid-day mediation is most helpful, for the reason I shared above. Even if you only have 20 minutes, you will feel the benefits.

Meditation can happen anywhere at any time but many add meditation into their daily routines. For me, my morning "meditation" is more about envisioning the day ahead and clarifying my desires and intentions. My mid-day practice is using the binaural beats. And nighttime, is more of a practice to calm and close out that day reflecting on the things I am grateful for from the day. I encourage you to create a routine that works for you, that you will stick with, There are also meditation classes (online or offline) you may want to join in to be part of a conscious community and deepen your understanding.

Mediation doesn't just have to be sitting or laying either. It can be doing activities that help quite your mind and activate being present. For many people it can be found in regular activities like vacuuming and ironing, or folding laundry. It could be walking in nature, sitting by the ocean or a stream listening to the sounds of the water and birds. It could be found in getting a massage, or running and exercising. Ultimately, being in a meditative state, is finding a place where you feel grounded, connected and calm.

## Detoxification

It is inevitable that toxins will enter our bodies through the environment and foods we eat, but we can minimize the amount of toxicity in our bodies by making cleaner lifestyle choices but also by having regular detoxification strategies in our life. Create habits that assist the body in elimination of toxins. The more toxic our bodies are the harder they are working, therefore the more tired and sluggish we feel. Too much toxicity in our bodies also makes us more susceptible to sickness.

Everyone feels great after doing aerobic exercise, our energy is up because our blood flow increases, our bodies get more oxygen, and hormonal changes happen. But in addition to that, aerobic exercise is a great way of helping your body eliminate toxins through sweat. It can accelerate the lymphatic system to move toxins out of the system more quickly.

I mentioned massages above. Massages aren't just a way to pamper ourselves but can be a regular part of our detoxification routine. I know it is definitely part of mine. Massages, especially deep tissue or lymphatic drainage, help by increasing circulation while the massage can help break up and free toxins that are lodged throughout the body. Reflexology is another helpful treatment to stimulate elimination. I get massages and reflexology weekly as my detox strategy to stay healthy and avoid getting sick but if I ever feel like I am getting sick, I go right to get a massage and usually stops before it sets in.

Natural detox teas, starting with green tea, are something else helpful to add into your daily routine. Many can help with stool elimination too. This is incredibly important. If you are not having regular bowel movements you are for sure holding too many toxins in your system. Adding greens and fiber are important to make sure you are regular. This is incredibly important and overlooked by many!

Sweating it out in sauna's can be useful too. Infrared saunas are really popular now because they are believed to help eliminate more toxins then traditional saunas.

A few more helpful detox strategies to add into your routine can be yoga, seaweed wraps, and breath work (can be found in many meditation classes) and using high quality liver detox supplements.

Be mindful that having things like alcohol, cigarettes, drugs, etc in your life can really tax your system with toxins a lot more than regular daily living. These types of toxic additions can stress the body, increase aging, sickness, and other diseases. If you are feeling really tired or sick often and have these types of substances in your life, you should consider removing them.

To get MORE of everything good out of life, everyone needs to be mindful of the role their physiological state plays in how they feel. This mindfulness makes people aware of what they are capable of doing. Just making some of the modifications I suggested can make a big difference in so many aspects. **Think of it as your energy management system; you want to make more deposits than withdraws for better long-term health, energy, upbeat moods, and mental clarity.** When you put all of that together, it leads to increased happiness, fulfillment, productivity, creativity, connectivity, and so much more!

## Journaling Prompts

1) How can you create a regular habit of treating your body as a temple? In using it as a place to show reverence and adoration, where can you direct that reverent energy? Where does that energy flow now, and how can you shift its direction?

2) In what areas of your overall wellness do you need to become more conscious of what your body needs?

3) In the past, have you pursued fitness or wellness? How can your approach to health focus more on your well-being than on society's definition of fitness?

## CHAPTER 5

# RESPONSIVE

## versus Reactive Life

Many years ago, I saw a movie called "The Way of the Peaceful Warrior". It was incredibly impactful. In the movie, there was a mentor and a student, and at one moment when the student was being triggered, the mentor said: "Fools react, warriors respond." I was blown away. It hit me in that moment that often, we go through life reacting rather than responding. I don't know about you, but I would much rather be a warrior than a fool.

I consciously made a decision that day to respond to life more often instead of reacting to it. I was already far into my path of spiritual discovery, which was making me more mindful and grounded, but I really wanted to master this concept.

Of course, choosing to be the warrior is one of the hardest things to master. So many of us have been subjected to reactionary examples throughout our lives, and it has become ingrained in who we are. Trying to master this is also an ongoing effort, because just when you think you have mastered it, the universe tests you with another challenge. But over time we can improve our relationship with these tests and see them exactly for what they are: tests. Mastering this skill is what that separates the good from great, the happy from sad, and the fulfilled from discontented.

In so many situations, people tend to lead with the ego (which is based on fear), needing to be right or to win in every situation rather than seeking to understand and resolve conflicts regardless of who is right. As my friend Michael Callejas says,

**"Your ego is NOT your amigo!"**

And it truly is not. Your ego is what keeps you stuck, making choices based on fear. People say to me all the time, "But wait! My ego is what makes me successful!" However, inner competitiveness is different from ego. Holding yourself accountable for your actions and pushing yourself forward is different from ego because ego can often come from a place of fear – whether that is fear of not being as good as you think you should be at something, fear that you are not as good as others, or fear that others won't like you.

In my quest to become more responsive than reactive, I discovered that I needed to continue to become more emotionally intelligent. Emotional intelligence is something I originally learned about in the mid-90's shortly after I graduated college. The way it breaks down is this: psychology is what goes on in the head (what we are thinking and the meaning we are giving things), and emotional intelligence is the heightened sense of self-awareness and ability to control the way that something happening makes you feel. And in a cycle between what's happening in our head and our emotions, we learn that we have the power to change what is going on in our mind and can almost instantly change how we are feeling.

When I learned about emotional intelligence, I was in the midst of my fitness career and I noticed that none of the emotional intelligence theories addressed the connection, or inner-connected cycle, between our physiological state and how we think, feel, and deal.

For example, you could be someone who is typically emotionally intelligent but if you haven't eaten and your blood sugar drops, you can become "hangry" and therefore impatient and difficult to deal with, which means your emotional intelligence is diminished due to your physiological state. The same thing could happen if you are tired or sick.

In essence, becoming more responsive means becoming more emotionally intelligent — which also means we need to become masterful of controlling our mindset and perspective, while also learning to assess and process our various emotional and physiological states. With these skills combined, when moments transpire where we are triggered or confronted, we can handle the situation better.

I recognized there were missing pieces in the puzzle of previous teaching of **how to become the best versions of ourselves.** Teaching emotional intelligence in its traditional sense wasn't enough, nor was psychology alone, nor were nutrition and physiology BUT connecting the dots between them all, along with a few other disciplines which I share as part of the MORE Method, needed to be part of the equation to truly get the best results of up-leveling who we are and what we are capable of. Connecting all of the dots of these various disciplines is how The MORE Method became my special formula and approach to helping people unlock their next level greatness.

So as you can see, in the previous chapters, I have laid the important foundation for you to become more responsive versus reactive because it truly is a layered approach.

From here on in this chapter, I will share with you a little more insight into emotional intelligence and the mindset shifts that took place for me in order to become more responsive than reactive even when triggered deeply. Let me preface again, this is not a path to perfection but a way to course correct more quickly when we fall down or make mistakes. I most certainly do not pass all of my tests, even with all of the training I have had. However, what I (and we) can do from this training that I am sharing with you is regroup more quickly, and fix my mistakes and choose better or differently in the future.

As my clients learn this information something always happens. They all will begin to see what they refer to as their "old self" and their "new self". For example, as they learn better ways about handling things in a situation, they can discern quickly and ask themselves, "Do I want to act like the old me or the new me?" Quite honestly, sometimes the ego will win the internal struggle and fall back to an old pattern, BUT there is progress to be proud of because now they will know and make statements like, "I know I should've handled it better but I couldn't help myself in the moment". They know the difference and can course-correct faster and play out mentally how they will handle it better the next time a similar situation transpires.

**Now the fine print: The limitation here is that many of us don't know how to deal with emotions because we were never taught how to. So many of us just don't know what we don't know. But if we are committed to learning, we can transform and up-level our lives quickly.**

I created the following mindset shifts as a strategy to teach you emotional intelligence in a way that you can quickly apply and even teach and share with others.

# MINDSET Shift 1

## Nothing Has Meaning Until You Give It Meaning

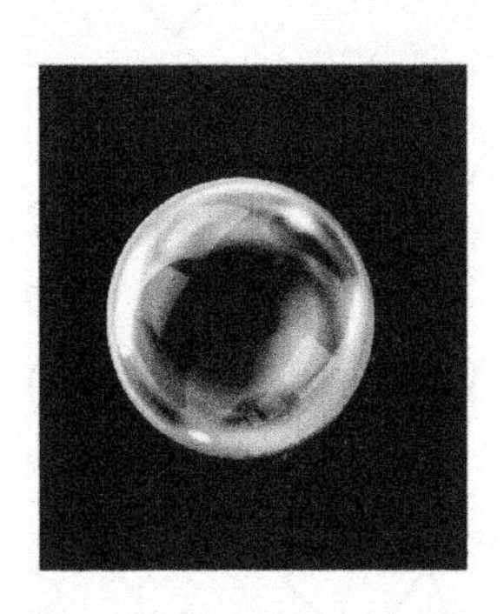

Nothing has
**MEANING**
until you give it
**MEANING**

The first time I heard this saying was shortly after my mother died 12 years ago. I was reading "Conversations with God" by Neale Donald Walsh and this notion changed my world. I re-read it multiple times. I put the book down and really took time to process how powerful this thought process was and how much it could change someone's life in an instant. I immediately thought about how this idea takes away anyone's ability to be a victim, because no matter what happened to you, you— and only YOU—have the power to give it meaning. The thoughts you choose impact how you feel, so you can choose to interpret a story in a way that frees you from anger or sadness, or you can prescribe a meaning that holds you captive and keeps you from happiness. It is our choice in every minute of every day.

Since my mom had just passed away at that time, it was like opening Pandora's box of childhood experiences and wounds. A little secret: bad memories never disappear when not dealt with. Instead, they sabotage your life and, for many, eventually create ongoing damage in relationships with others. It was an interesting time, processing these suppressed memories (many hurtful and traumatic), but this new perspective gave me the power. I realized all of these experiences from my childhood that could be seen as hurtful were actually helpful and were propelling me to become the woman I needed to be today. I realized these experiences became my training ground for success.

We have the power to go back to every story in our lives and change them to something positive. Immediately. Today.

I know, I know, some of you are thinking, "No way Jen, that person cheated on me, or stole from me, or abused me." The list can go on and on. And I get it, there are a lot of crappy experiences we go through, but giving those stories power still keeps you from *your* power. So, change it to serve you. Change it to help you grow. Forgive whoever wronged you—because the only prisoner to that anger is you.

There is an old Buddhist saying, "Would you rather be right or happy?" I always laugh when I ask this question in groups because there will always be people that say, "Well, I am happy when I am right." Those people are operating with their ego in the driver's seat and need to begin a big shift.

I learned that lesson myself when I started my handbag company. I had incredible goals for the company, and there were a lot of milestones I wanted to reach. One of my biggest goals was to license my company, because I knew it would help me reach my financial goals. So when I was introduced to one of the top leaders in the handbag and accessories industry, I saw a huge opportunity. Just looking at the office spaces he operated and the lifestyle he lived, I knew I wanted to be a part of what he was doing. I mean, he was working with brands like Calvin Klein and Eli Tahari. I wanted to be in that echelon.

At that stage of my life, I couldn't imagine being any luckier when I had that meeting. But that admiration and desire led me to make decisions that weren't of the highest consciousness.

When I met the guy, I instantly got the intuition that he was a bit shady. His operation seemed somewhat unethical, and he hit on me almost immediately after meeting me, since we were both married. In my gut I felt that working with him was probably not the best business decision. But my ego wanted that deal so bad. I wanted to be able to say that I was part of that world. So I didn't listen to my intuition. I listened to my ego.

Within just a few years, the man was stealing from all of his brands. He would take from one brand to pay the other brand, and his glamorous façade came crumbing down. It was like a house of cards with all of the other brands he was working with. I learned that he had been stealing from me all along, skimming off of my royalties.

This put me in a really compromising position. The whole situation could have destroyed my brand. When I was no longer working with him, I went from receiving decreased royalties from several retailers to only receiving checks from Avon (which still turned out to be a great deal later on). But it put me in a bad financial position overnight, because we had heavily invested in that growth, and created a lot of overhead with employees and other financial obligations.

At that point, I was confronted with a really big decision. When I realized what had happened, and I realized that I wasn't the only brand this was happening to, I needed to decide how to move forward. Was I going to sue him, or was I going to just keep pushing for growth on my own? I eventually decided not to sue and moved on.

The reason I want to share this story is because it's important to learn how we're spending our energy. If we're spending our energy looking backward in a negative, toxic place, we could really be destroying our future success.

When I evaluated my situation, I had to recognize first of all that many of the other, bigger brands he was working with had a lot more money than I did, so they were going to be out in front of it. I also realized that I would have to spend the next three to five years of my life looking back through old emails and files if I wanted to start a legal case. But I believed that God gave me enough creativity and resourcefulness to keep moving forward. I learned the lessons that were presented in that situation and used it as an opportunity for growth.

For me, the biggest lesson from that situation was that I need to listen to my intuition. While this is a lesson that we often know already, it sometimes takes a tough experience to remind you not to doubt your gift of intuition.

Now, I put that lesson to use every day. Ever since that situation, I really do put a lot of power into my intuition. Even when my logic is thinking or hoping something different, I put a lot of faith into what my intuition is telling me.

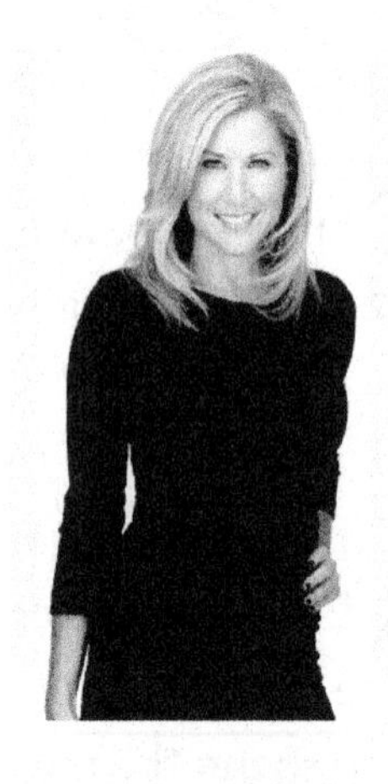

YOU are the Director of your life.

Too often we give our power away. We lose our authentic-self in other people's projections and expectations.

We minimize ourselves to gain the approval of others only to realize later in life their approval nor opinions were worth anything of value on our life journey.

But today, and every day, that can change once we step back into our power because we can be the writer, director and producer of our story - Every. Single. Day.

The excuses are the lies we keep rehearsing to play small and rob us of our potential.

Rewrite the old stories that still hold you captive. Give them different meaning. Give them meaning that serves you. That expands you. And most importantly, frees you.

Play the movie that you want to live out in your head. Envision it. Feel it. Then BECOME it.

We are the meaning makers of our lives. We are in control of the meanings we chose to give every life experience. When we do that, we can stop reacting so much and start responding.

What stories have been running and ruining your life? And how can you change them now to empower your life? Re-write these stories. All of them. They are your key to freedom and the foundation and ongoing mindset to get MORE of everything you desire in life.

# MINDSET Shift 2

## The Only Thing We Have Control Of in the World Is Our Perspective

I know this belief can freak out a lot of control freaks, but it is true. The sooner we understand that, the more we can feel comfort in the power of our perspective and become capable of seeing multiple perspectives to understand other people.

How we view the world is based on our perspectives. Often, we have one perspective in any given situation, which means we are usually lacking empathy and compassion. A limited view causes us to be judgmental of others, which also means we struggle with deeply connected, fulfilling relationships. This is not a good trait, and no way to get MORE of everything good in life.

The more we can train ourselves to see multiple perspectives, the more successful relationships we can nurture. Mastering multiple perspectives creates the best leaders, parents, and communicators.

An eye-opening exercise is to stop and think before projecting your perspectives on how something played out, and instead ask someone else how they viewed something. The more you do this, the more you will realize how even when we live through the same experiences, we view them differently. You can really see this unfold with adult siblings and their views of their childhoods.

Many years ago, I had an experience that taught me about perspective in a surprising way. I had been dating a guy, who we'll call Phil, for a little while, and he invited me to go to a party with him. The party wasn't happening for another couple of months, so I made a mental note about it. I didn't put it on my calendar—quite honestly, I wasn't sure if we would even be dating still at that point.

Now, here's something you should know about me: I'm a huge Eagles fan. I go to many of the games; it's one of my favorite things to do. So wouldn't you know that the day of the party Phil invited me to also happened to be the same night as a playoff game. I had been really looking forward to that game, so I offered to get Phil a ticket so we could go to the game together instead of the party.

Well, Phil was furious with me. He felt like I was choosing the game over him. But I didn't know that at first, because he wasn't willing to communicate with me. Instead of talking through it with me in the moment, he started playing games. He wouldn't respond to me, he acted childish, and behaved like he was throwing a temper tantrum. When the night of the game arrived, he wouldn't even respond to me until the next day.

In order to get the situation smoothed out, I had to recognize that getting mad right back at him wouldn't help anything. I needed to figure out what meaning he was giving the situation, because I wasn't really sure. I just knew that I was annoyed because he wasn't understanding that the Eagles game was very meaningful to me, and it felt like he was being irrational but in his perspective he thought I wasn't prioritizing the relationship.

The moment I realized this was so profound to me. I finally understood that, while I really believed that I was right, he also believed that he was right. And in the middle was an understanding that we had to get to in order to have empathy and compassion for each other. Would that understanding have changed the decision I made? Probably not. But I think I would have been more compassionate in how I handled the situation. I could have been more affirming in the words I chose, assuring him that my decision had nothing to do with how I felt about the relationship.

That experience with Phil really taught me how many relationships have these kinds of moments. It's so important to bring emotional intelligence and empathetic communication skills to the table with every relationship we cultivate. Both Phil and I believed we were right, just as many people do. And once we understood each other's point of view, we were able to see each other's perspective and feel less hurt by the experience.

That's where most people fall apart. They don't even know that they don't know. And so, in order to get MORE of everything good out of life, we have to learn how to share our playbook with each other. We have to say, "Here's how I'm feeling and this is why I'm feeling it. I would love to understand how you're feeling so that we can operate with each other better."

Keep in mind, when you are able to see multiple perspectives, you may not (and do not have to) agree with someone else's point of view. But you can respect their perception because it is coming from their previous life experiences.

**Letting go of the need to be right and seeking to understand by seeing through the lens of other perspectives instantly puts you into a place of power over your emotions, allows you to be triggered less, and helps you stay calm more.**

In your MORE Method Journal, challenge yourself to think about situations that triggered you to be judgmental or upset in the past and re-evaluate them with your new power of perspective. Step into the shoes of the other people involved and challenge yourself to think about how they may have viewed the situation. Let go of your ego in this exercise or you will *never* master this skill. Going forward, challenge yourself to see other people's perspectives—it really broadens our interpretations of the world around us!

# MINDSET Shift 3

## Hurt People Hurt People, Happy People Don't

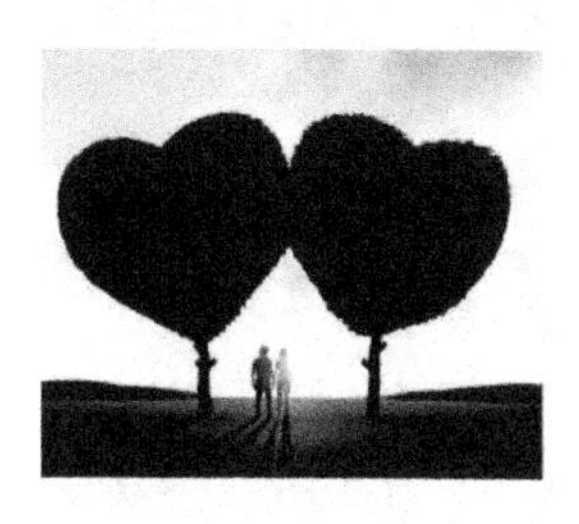

**HURT**
People Hurt People,
**HAPPY**
People Don't

Psychological projections happen all day, every day. The definition of psychological projection is "a defense mechanism in which the human ego defends itself against unconscious impulses or qualities denying their existence in themselves while attributing them to others. Psychological projections involve projecting undesirable feelings or emotions onto someone else, rather than admitting to or dealing with the unwanted feelings."

I have been repeating the mantra above to my daughters since they were very little. When I first heard it as an adult, I wanted every child to hear this so they didn't allow other people's pain to become theirs. The "bully" is in pain—that could have saved me a lot of pain and shame in back in school. But unfortunately, it doesn't stop in school. Many adults continue the patterns well into their adult lives without even realizing it. Someone's pain ends up damaging everyone else.

When my daughters started middle school, a time when bullying is at its height, I told them something I wish I had known when I was their age. I said, "Listen, hurt people hurt people, happy people don't. If someone is being mean at school, they are probably going through something at home. You can have compassion and walk away. But don't pick up the stones they throw, because if you do, you end up filling your backpack with other people's stones and it becomes heavier and heavier as you age." My girls' eyes grew as I shared this with them because they didn't even like carrying an empty wrapper of something. They thought of a carrying a heavy backpack, all day, every day was not something they wanted a part of. Interestingly enough, they got their first test the first week of 5th grade.

Madison and Morgan had only been in fifth grade for a few days when one of their friends fell prey to another girl in the class, who we will call Sara. Their friend is a lot pretty shy, and Sara began bullying her in the schoolyard. But because of how I programmed my daughters, Madison's first response was to say, "Sara, we live in a drama-free zone. You need to keep your drama out of our space." She continued, saying, "You can be our friend again when you learn to be a better friend."

When Madison told me the story, I was so proud of her for using what she's learned at home. What was especially interesting to me was that she didn't just say, "You can't be our friend anymore," but rather, "You can be our friend again when you learn to be a better friend." Now, I taught her that we live in a drama-free zone, but I had never heard the second part before. I asked her where she learned it. She said to me, "Mom, you taught me that hurt people hurt people. And Sara's parents are going through a divorce right now. I think that Sara is just in pain. So I didn't want to tell her she couldn't be our friend again forever. But I figured when she was out of pain, and maybe when her parents weren't going through a divorce, she would become a better friend."

It was so powerful. Because kids just get this consciousness so well. Madison was so compassionate when she understood that hurt people hurt people. And she gave Sara an opportunity to become a better version of herself, recognizing at a young age that people aren't necessarily their behavior. Sometimes people act the way they do because there's something else going on in their lives. And that is a huge thing that we need to understand.

**Sometimes people are not being the best versions of themselves, not because of who they are, but because of what they are going through.**

Madison taught me such a great way to articulate that kind of circumstance. I'm so proud of her, because throughout the school year, Sara watched how Madison and Morgan treated their friends. And now that she has emerged on the other side of that struggle she was dealing with, Sara is now one of Madison and Morgan's best friends. She was just going through a tough time and didn't know how to express her emotions.

I often think about what might have happened if my girls had just cut her off. What if they had bullied her right back? What path would she have gone on? I don't know the answer to that, but I don't think it would have been as wonderful as it is for her today.

We all need to be conscious of understanding that hurt people hurt people. Instead of mirroring back their behaviors and potentially hurting them more, we need to learn to be more compassionate. Maybe we need to remove ourselves from that person's life or take some distance. But we do still need to ask ourselves: "Is this something that's changing who they are for the moment? Is it something I can assist them with to help them get through a hard time?"

Once we recognize other peoples' behaviors as projections of their own unhappiness, we can shift from emotions—like anger and resentment—to emotions like compassion and empathy. Please know, I am not saying that it is okay to abuse, bully or cast your stones on others. But once we can understand the *why,* we can stop thinking it is about things in terms of how much something is about us when someone is acting out. We can let the stones they throw lay on the ground and walk away with our own inner calm.

We can also choose to engage when someone casts their stones at us, if it is someone we care about deeply. Our first instinct may be to feel defensive and possibly to fight back, or put the other person in their place, so to speak. But those reactions come from the ego and only serves to bring us to a lower level. However, if you care about the person, this can be an opportunity to help them—we just need to approach the situation from a place of compassion and empathy. It can be a teachable moment. For example, if it's a close friend or an intimate partner and they say or do something we perceive as hurtful, instead of just attacking them and trying to blame or shame them, calmly say something like, "Hey, I am sure you didn't mean to but that wasn't very nice. Is everything okay with you?"

Starting with, "I am sure you didn't mean to..." alleviates the feeling that they are being attacked, so they will feel safer to share. Following with a question like, "is everything okay with you?" is expressing your care for their well-being. Ideally this opens a dialogue for the person to share what's going on. The posture needed in these conversations always comes from a place of love, despite what the other person is doing.

If they are being too difficult to deal with, you can excuse yourself from the conversation until they are in a better place. This is not opportunity to storm out the door and say something passive aggressive. This is a time to say something like, "I am sorry something is obviously bothering you, and I would love to help, but I will not be a punching bag. I am here to listen when you are ready to share, but I expect respect in the process." This expresses your care and concern but also creates clear boundaries of how you expect to be treated.

There is a Buddhist saying, "If you can't help others, at least do not harm them." So often, we snap back at people when they cast their stones, and if they are already in pain about something else it only compounds their problem. We can harm people more than we know, or we can heal them with simple acts of kindness. With love, we can heal them even more. But we are always walking around so guarded by our own fears that we miss these magical opportunities.

The truth is, when we help others heal, we also heal. It is one of the most gratifying experiences we can encounter consistently. The more our society can become emotionally intelligent, the more we can all thrive collectively. The more we lead with kindness and compassion, the MORE we can get everything we desire from life.

# MINDSET Shift 4

## Our Expectations of Others Cause Our Own Self-Inflicted Pain

There is a famous quote from Danny Wilson, "Life is easy. We make it hard." And in many ways, for the general population reading this, I would agree with his sentiment. It's hard for me to witness on a daily basis how many people cause their own pain with the expectations they create for others to think like them, act like them, and feel like them. When someone cannot live up to those expectations, they become mad at the other person.

What's even worse is these are most often **unexpressed expectations** that no one else has agreed to. It's really crazy when we break it down because essentially, we are all supposed to go around the world like mind readers. Under these conditions we would all need to make ourselves consistently unhappy to constantly fill the voids of others to make them happy.

My friend Jenny is a great example of this. Around the time that my children and Jenny's first child were the same age and were very young, she decided that she wanted to have another child. Jenny was extremely committed to her career and she came by it honestly. Her dad was a really successful businessman, and she worshipped her dad and looked up to his accomplishments. She really carried an immense sense of responsibility and desire to be successful like him.

When she told me she wanted another child, I said to her, "Are you sure you want to have another child already? You know, you're already feeling overwhelmed with the first child and your career." Still, she insisted that she was ready. But, when she had her second child, she became overwhelmed and felt very frustrated that she was doing a lot of things, but nothing right. She decided to quit her job to be a stay at home mom, and I cautioned her that she may not find that to be the best solution for her personality. She said, "Well, I just feel like I'm failing at everything."

She quit her job, and very quickly, she became very unhappy after work every day. She was complaining a lot more about little things and she started getting sick all the time. She complained about her husband, who was going golfing and doing other things he wanted after work every day because he didn't want to be home.

So I said to her, "I really think you need to re-think this career strategy, because you're becoming a different person and it's really overwhelming." She really got aggravated and angry at me for saying that, and continued her pattern of complaining more and more, being focused on little things that were really nothing that became big things to her.

Still, Jenny kept asking for my advice, and I'd say to her, "I really believe you quitting your career is part of this because you're not feeling fulfilled."

Eventually, I just stopped giving her advice. Every piece of advice I could give to her, she got mad at me for saying anyway. As a result, I started distancing myself as her friend.

I never shamed her, and I wasn't mean to her. I just started distancing myself. And the more I distanced myself, the angrier she became at me. About two years into this experience, maybe even a little bit longer, her husband reached out to me. He said, "Listen, Jenny is in a really bad place. I really would love if you could reach out to her."

So, a few days after that, Jenny texted me asking for a book recommendation, explaining that she was in a bad state. I thought, "Yes, this is awesome. She's finally hitting rock bottom and searching for ways to climb out of the hole that she created." So, I not only sent her the name of a book, I sent her a name of three books, a video for this movie called *The Shift* by Wayne Dyer, and a meditation link.

Jenny never responded. Then the next day, she says, "Can you please meet me?" So, as a working mom of two young girls, I dropped everything that I planned that next night to meet her for dinner. We got to the restaurant, and I was barely even in my seat when Jenny said to me, "You are the worst friend ever."

I sat in shock at first. She said, "I texted you last night or two nights ago to ask you for the name of a book. And I told you I was in a bad place." And I immediately grabbed my phone to say, "I texted you back. Didn't you see? I texted three books, the name of a movie and a meditation link." And then she walloped me with the real issue: "Any good friend would have known to pick up the phone and call."

"No, that's not the truth," I said. "Because when I ask for something, I'm literally asking for what I'm asking for. I'm not asking someone to read between the lines of what I'm asking and what I really need."

I felt set up and manipulated. And this is something that people do to each other all of the time. So I said to her, "Jenny, you know what's interesting is that you need me right now because of the dysfunctional and crazy childhood that I had. I have all these resiliency skills; I have all this knowledge and wisdom of how to get out of a bad place. And you grew up in this amazing, perfect childhood, where your mom was home baking cookies and making snacks for you after school every day. And you traveled the world. And you went to the best schools, and everything was just perfect. So, you don't have the same skills as me. But you're asking me to think like you and think like me at the same exact time, which is really impossible. Because I haven't walked in your shoes, I can't think like you, I can only think like me. And if I text somebody and ask for a question or a resource, I'm literally just asking for the resource. And if I wanted to talk to them, I would pick up the phone and call them."

I realized that that was her breakthrough moment. She said, "I don't even know who I am anymore."

I wasn't afraid to be truthful to her in that moment. I kept in mind that my truth isn't her truth. It's just my perspective. But I wasn't willing to placate her like her other friends were because she wasn't able to be the best version of herself that way. And I wasn't afraid of the conflict. What Jenny was doing is what a lot of people do—projecting all of her ill feelings about her life on to me and making them my fault. And, like many people do, she was manipulating me as a friend into having to behave a certain way to think like her, act like her, and be like her, which is completely impossible. This is one of the biggest things that we do to each other in relationships and in friendships, and it is highly damaging.

I briefly spoke about expectations earlier, but let's break down the three types of expectations we hold even further.

First, there are expectations for your own life. Here, you can and should have high standards for how your life plays out and how others treat you. But you are responsible for this, not others. You have the ability to constantly make choices to evaluate if people and circumstances align and support with the expectations you have for your own life.

Second is the unexpressed expectations which we have discussed above. These are the expectations that cause our own pain and suffering. So what happens when people in our life aren't meeting our expectations? Well, we can either 1) change our expectations and accept people for who they are where they are or 2) wean or eliminate them out of our lives.

1) In changing our expectations and accepting people for who they are, we are accepting self-

responsibility and exercising a lot of emotional intelligence. Let's be honest, there are some people we can't, or shouldn't, just remove from our lives just because we can't manage our expectations properly.

Accepting people for who they are and where they are is actually the highest form of respect. The more we do this, the MORE we can appreciate many people of many walks of life because we move out of constant judgment.

2) Distancing or eliminating certain people can be a good self-preservation strategy when coming from the right place. This can be a bit different in the dynamic of friendships and family. Too often people feel like they need to make someone feel in the wrong when they decide a relationship is not good for them, and we simply don't need to do that. That falls into the "causing harm to others" bucket. If someone directly asks you about the distance you can either say something like, "I have been really busy and need to focus on some other priorities right now," or even use it as an opportunity to have a productive conversation about issues that may exist. But giving someone the silent treatment to hurt them isn't the way to go.

The third type of expectation is expressed and agreed upon expectations. This is what should really be happening in every single relationship. If not, we are essentially asking people to be mind-readers and then get mad at people when they let us down because they can't read minds. This technique is used with all masterful communicators and it should be a goal for everyone. When you are in relationship (any kind of relationship dynamic) and expectations arise, we should clearly express them to others. Now, the other person does not need to agree upon them. This is where a dialogue happens and possibly even a compromise. Or perhaps the other person cannot or will not agree upon the expectations, then we have a moment of "truth", to decide how we would like to move forward from there. Or if everything goes well, and expectations are expressed and agreed upon, and one doesn't live up to their promise, disappointment is a valid and a new conversation has to begin from there. But remember, when communicating your expectation that you want someone to agree upon them, make sure they tell you what they are agreeing upon in their own words. SO often what we say, isn't NOT what someone is hearing. This is another great technique to use to enhance your communication skills.

Learning about expectations is ultimately about learning how to manage our own expectations of others. If you find that everyone keeps letting you down, and instead of doing work within yourself, you just cut people out of your life and place blame on everyone else, then you haven't learned from this book. That's the easy way out. If you are seeing that you are the common denominator of something negative, the work has to come from within. Highly emotionally intelligent people are in harmony with most people because they have learned to take responsibility for themselves and their expectations, communicate effectively, while having a high level of acceptance for others. When we communicate our expectations of others and take into account their own expectations, we can prevent heartache and give ourselves MORE of the things we desire in life.

# MINDSET Shift 5

## There Is Power In Pause and Space

People who have reactive personalities usually do not take time to pause and process what they are thinking and feeling to reframe and respond more responsibly. The reason I use the word "responsibly" is because when we react versus respond, we are usually acting irresponsibly with our emotions, and therefore will choose to say or do things that can cause more damage than good in a situation.

**We must learn to:**

1) **Pause**
2) **Process**
3) **Reflect to Reframe**
4) **Responsibly Respond**

When you do this four-step process, you will become better in every aspect of your life. You will be a better leader, partner, and parent because you will diminish the number of emotional explosions. Now, let's expand on what that four-step process actually entails.

1) **Pause:** When you are feeling triggered or overwhelmed, pause and take deep breaths. Think calming thoughts. Usually this is thinking about something or someone you love. Then ask yourself, "If I respond now, will it be of my highest self?" If you are feeling fired up, the answer is probably, "No." If the answer is no, it is completely responsible to say, "I am going to need to take some time to process before I respond." I often also add, "If I respond right now you are probably not going to like what I have to say, and I won't either because I won't be the best version of myself." I have incredible respect for people when they do that because they are showing a high level of self-awareness and emotional restraint. That is the quality found in some on the greatest leaders.

2) **Process:** Taking time to process how you are feeling about something. This means gaining time and space from the person or problem in order to reevaluate after the emotional charge of

the situation has dissipated. Once the emotional charge passes, we can often see things differently and will gain a different perspective.

3) **Reflect to Reframe:** This leads us to the next step, where we challenge ourselves to reframe the situation. Take control of the scenario by seeing it differently. Ask questions like, "How can I approach/see this differently?" or "What might the other person be needing or feeling that's causing this underlying issue?" You may also want to ask yourself, "What do I really want and need out of this situation? How can everyone get their needs met in this situation?" Creating a list of reframing questions that you use as litmus test is a very useful strategy.

4) **Responsibly Respond:** Responsibly responding means that you have cooled off a bit, reflected and reframed and have put your ego in check for the intention of a productive conversation. Not a conversation to be right, but a conversation seeking resolution where both parties feel good or at minimum okay about how things went.

This method of conflict resolution is useful at home, work, or even when you are just running into roadblocks of your own making. We are so conditioned as a society to find the quickest solution that we often forget the power in pausing. Use the exercise above to fully embrace and harness all of the resources you can find when you pause.

I used this exercise myself with a friend I'll call Brandi. Brandi has such an incredible heart, but she's had experiences in her life that she hasn't been able to deal with. I noticed that Brandi self-medicated with excessive alcohol on a regular basis.

One night, I invited Brandi to attend an important event as my guest. There were a lot of high-profile people there, so it was kind of a big deal. Brandi arrived at six o'clock, but she was completely intoxicated. She also brought with her another person, who was very abrupt and apt to complain. It was a disaster waiting to happen.

It was still cocktail hour, and dinner wouldn't be served for quite a while, but Brandi was getting hungry. Because she was so intoxicated, she started making a scene. Of course, this commotion was happening in the middle of an interview with one of the most legendary football coaches of the NFL. At that point, the CEO of the company I was partnered with approached me and said, "You need to ask Brandi to leave. This is absolutely disruptive and disrespectful."

I knew Brandi was already being difficult; with her being so out of it, my asking her to leave would add even more fuel to the fire. So another man from the organization asked her to leave, causing her to make even more of a scene.

Eventually the CEO escorted her to leave. I was humiliated. She was my guest; she was there because of me. I was embarrassed because she had caused such a scene, and she had disrupted the entire event for everyone attending.

The next morning, I woke up to several missed calls and text messages from Brandi. The messages were all aggressive, attacking both me and the organization. She said the event wasn't good, the food wasn't on time, etc. And not once did she take responsibility for the fact that she had been highly intoxicated and created a scene.

I didn't answer the messages at first. Eventually, I messaged her back and said, "Brandi, I am not in a position to respond to you right now. Whatever I say to you will not be of the highest version of myself. I need to emotionally process how I'm feeling right now before I can respond to you, because what I say will not be productive at all at this moment."

It took me about five days for the anger I had toward her to cool off. Brandi hated having to wait for my response, because it kept her in that fight within her head, planning what she was going to say to me. But I can only be responsible for myself. I knew that I could not respond in a good way in that state, so I waited.

When I finally came back to the conversation with Brandi, I was able to address it in a less reactive way. What I had to tell Brandi was that I knew she was a very good person, but I was concerned that her need to drink at events was causing her to be a lesser version of herself. By that point, the conversation was well-received by both of us. This was because I was able to be calm in the way I handled it. I started the dialogue by complimenting her, telling her that I believe she's a really good person instead of attacking her. Then I calmly offered her my perception of why I was concerned about her behavior.

By taking those days to pause and collect myself, we had a very different conversation than we would have had if I'd talked to her the very next morning. Because I waited and handled it in a responsible way, Brandi and I actually became closer through this conflict. Our trust grew because I didn't attack her in the way she expected me to.

We need to take the time necessary to be the best version of ourselves when we respond to conflict. It's so important to pause so that we can be as productive with our actions as possible. **During that pause, we get a chance to reflect and focus on the root of our feelings, not just the situation that happened.**

Now, I do want to make an important distinction. There's a big difference between taking space to process and withdrawing to punish someone. They are very different actions. Withdrawing to punish someone is pure manipulation, whereas pausing and asking for space is done with the intention of coming back as the best person you can be to handle the situation. It's important to communicate to the other person that you're taking a pause and why you are taking that pause. Because if you don't communicate your intentions, it will feel to the other person like you're withdrawing from them as a punishment. And people who withdraw to manipulate are not setting up a good foundation for a beneficial, compassionate long-term outcome.

When we give ourselves the time and space to bring out our best selves, we are more effective in getting MORE of the things we desire in life.

# MINDSET Shift 6

## There Is a Lesson In Everything That Happens to Us

I believe that no matter what happens, we can gain wisdom from each and every situation—especially the ones that really stink. When you shift your mindset to realize this, nothing can actually happen in vain. We can find grace in gratitude and feel empowered and strengthened from challenging experiences. This ties directly into the idea that "nothing has meaning until you give it meaning."

My father just passed away a few weeks ago as I write this. Anyone who has lost a parent knows what a challenging experience that is. I was at his house the day before and I told him I would be back the next day to bring him more of the tomato soup he liked. As I was on my way to his house that next day, my plans got derailed because my daughters needed to be picked up unexpectedly. I changed my course and headed to pick them up, thinking I would just bring the soup to my dad the next day because I needed to get back home and get ready for a play I was seeing that night. Everything seemed so normal, until it wasn't anymore.

Unfortunately, that night while I was at the play, I found out that my dad fell. I beat myself up immediately, thinking, "What if I had brought the soup earlier like I intended to? Would that have somehow changed the course of what have happened?" A million scenarios played out in my head.

After he fell, there was a domino effect. He suffered from complications in the hospital, and almost two weeks later, he was gone. This was a life experience where it was hard to find the positive or the lesson. This just plain sucked. I began to turn to sadness and despair until I remembered this valuable lesson—a lesson that we all logically know, but often don't put a lot of severe weight in. The lesson was to never take for granted someone who will always be there tomorrow, because tomorrow is not promised. I learned from my father's passing to live everyday like it can be your own or someone else's last day. This was a lesson affirmed the hard way, but it sure brought a profound shift in my way of living— and for that I am grateful, because I will live each day and moment to the fullest without taking it for granted. But I may not have understood this lesson if I didn't believe that everything that happens to us can bring a lesson we need to learn. Because I understood this, I was able to find something positive in such a dark time. The more we seek the lessons in every situation, the MORE we'll get everything we desire in life.

# MINDSET Shift 7

## There Is Power in Conflict

When I am speaking and teaching this topic at events, I always ask the crowd, "How many of you avoid conflict?" Almost everyone raises their hand in the room, every time.

Then I ask, "How many of you ever thought of conflict as an incredible way to build a deeper connection with someone?" I *may* get a few hands up, but it is mostly crickets and people nervously looking to see who raised their hands. It's so powerful to see the societal programming around the belief that conflict is bad and should be avoided at all costs. When I suggest a new belief, that maybe it could be a good thing to build depth in relationships, people look at me like, "What did she just say? How is that even possible?" But as we have learned in this book, once the belief shifts, so does how we feel about it, and how we approach it.

I believe conflict, when dealt with properly and in an emotionally intelligent way, deepens trust and intimacy in any relationship. There is a lot to be said for relationships that are challenged, and even more to be said of two people who decide to go through the uncomfortable stuff because they care about the relationship too much to just throw it away like day-old bagels. Sadly though, more people than not are so afraid of conflict that they dispose of friendships or relationships because they don't have the tools for productive conflict. But when we see the positive results that can come from productive conflict, we can approach these situations with less fear and more excitement to get to know the other person better and share an experience together that deepens the relationship.

**We are seeking to understand others instead of seeking to be right.**

When we avoid conflict and don't deal with things as they come, resentment builds until someone explodes. Ironically, the explosive moment usually comes after something insignificant because the little things piled on top of each other for so long.

The better we are at dealing with things as they transpire, the better we feel about the people around us. Speaking our ego-free truth to others makes us better communicators, more emotionally connected, and more authentic in our relationships.

**NOTE: Remember, your "truth" isn't THE truth, it's just YOUR "truth." The more we seek to resolve conflict successfully, the MORE fulfilling our relationships will be, and the MORE we will get what we desire in life.**

# MINDSET Shift 8

## The Health of Our Relationships Is Directly Connected to Our Success and Happiness

When we were growing up, we often were told to go to school, get good grades, get a good job, and work really hard and then you will be successful and happy. Not nearly as often do we hear something like, "Go to school, learn how to connect with people, create great relationships, nurture those relationships, and stay away from toxic relationships because they will quickly destroy your happiness and your best efforts at being successful at work." As a matter of fact, many people follow the first piece of advice, and as they get older and they find that they put their work first, believing that's more important. They realize they didn't consistently nurture their relationships, or they stay in relationships that don't support or fulfill them and then find themselves in in the throes of disruption.

In the wildly successful book *Lean In* by Sheryl Sandberg, the loudest message I heard was that she wouldn't be where she is without the support of her amazing husband. When you read between the lines of her story, you will hear, "Hey ladies, if you want to "Lean In" and be successful *and* have a family, be very careful about who you choose to marry."

When we are in thriving intimate relationships, our happiness and careers thrive. That seems obvious, right? But I witness so many people ignoring this fact—stuck in flailing or failing relationships that constantly make them stressed, unhappy and distracted at work. They are never allowing their full potential to be accessed. I have been in some relationships to experience this truth and know first hand the destruction it can cause. I meet so many young, incredible people who stay in toxic romances and I beg them from my experiences to see the tethers it creates in their futures.

This isn't just about intimate relationships, though. This is about the health of ALL relationships.

**Emotionally Intelligent people prioritize and aim for relationship harmony.**

Whether it's family, friends, or co-workers, the healthier your relationships are, the less stress and toxicity you have in your life. Becoming a masterful communicator and becoming highly aware of yourself and others helps you to navigate people and relationships in ways that add greater fulfillment to your life. These abilities also eliminate many of the disruptions and distractions that hold you back from a greater life. They apply all of the lessons you have learned thus far to navigate even the more difficult people. Imagine being able to go through life barely affected by relationship drama. Well, that's the goal to aim for, and is achievable by applying and practicing all of the lessons you have learned here.

To get MORE of everything you desire in life, prioritize the health of your relationships. Use the tips and strategies in this book to help enhance them and remove the toxic ones that are constantly derailing your best efforts. In essence, detox the drainers and increase the enhancers. I know sometimes this is easier said than done, especially if you love someone. It's important to love yourself more.

# MINDSET Shift 9

## Whatever Triggers Us is Not Yet Healed

Here is another lesson from my relationship with Phil. One day Phil and I we were having a discussion, but in the middle of the conversation, Phil's voice volume and tone changed. His volume increased and his tone triggered something in me—it felt almost as if someone was pinching the sensitive back of my arm. It was the type of trigger that you want to *react* to quickly and fiercely for retaliation.

His tone triggered me because it reminded me of the voice that my dad would use when I was younger. And instead of Phil getting my attention like he desired, I felt I had two options: I could shut down and do nothing or I could push back and really react. Instead, I took the secret hidden option number three: in that moment, I took a deep breath, and asked myself why it was triggering me so much.

"I know you're trying to get my attention for something," I said. "I know you need me to hear you. But I can't when you speak to me in this tone of voice because it is triggering me. It is same tone that my dad took when I was younger. And, while I know that's not your fault, if you want to communicate with me effectively and get my attention, this is not the way to do it. I would prefer you to speak to me in a tone that is more nurturing and softer. And I know you want what you want, and I want what I want, so I'm trying to teach you how to get to that place."

He was shocked because he had never really had a conversation like this where someone actually pointed out their triggers. Nobody had ever told him how to communicate effectively with them.

But more importantly, I knew in that moment that some of the childhood stuff that I thought was resolved within me, wasn't. I knew it wasn't resolved because if it was, I wouldn't have reacted with such anger and resentment. This was something I needed to reflect and work on because I didn't want it to hide deep inside of me anymore.

The best thing to do when we have triggers is look them dead on and deal with it.

We can imagine this process like riding a hot air balloon. Every hot air balloon begins on the ground. This stage is symbolic of the beginning of the journey of your evolution. It's the awakening moment; the moment when you're at your lowest point and decide that you want a change.

The only way to get to the next level in the hot air balloon is to remove some of the sandbags. The sandbags are symbolic of your "stuff." You need to remove some of this "stuff"—the beliefs, behaviors, and unhealed trauma keeping you from being your best self—in order to get to the next level. And when you get rid of these sandbags, the hot air balloon begins to rise as you personally begin to rise.

Eventually, you find yourself hovering somewhere new. You get to see a new perspective of what the world around you looks like. Maybe you live in New York City, and you're used to seeing all of the buildings. But when you take off, you start to see how many trees are in Central Park. You might say, "Wow, this is a new perspective. I never knew how many trees were in Central Park. This is so cool!"

Pretty soon, you get used to seeing the world through these new eyes. And most people eventually get bored. So you begin to venture into your **next stage of evolution**.

But again, the only way to get to that next level in your evolution is to get rid of more sandbags. So what beliefs, behaviors, and unhealed trauma are keeping you from getting to the next level? You have to choose which things you're going to take out so you can rise again. This is a process. It's a journey of evolution. At every stage, you need to continue to evaluate what things are keeping you down and begin to remove them. Otherwise you'll stay exactly where you are, hovering in the same place forever.

In order to evolve, you've got to be able to do the work. It's heavy lifting those sandbags out. Sometimes it's hard work. But it's worth it for the new view and the perspective that you're going to gain. Because every time you move to a new height, you gain a new perspective and become more aware of your surroundings. And the new perspective is always better than the last perspective. It won't necessarily get easier as the process continues. But the work is worth it.

A lot of people struggle to get off the ground in the hot air balloon because they don't understand the value of doing the heavy lifting to get the first few sandbags out. Don't be afraid to do the work, look within, and let go. Don't be afraid of losing control, because the excitement of the change is greater than the fear. Be excited for the unknown rather than fearful of it.

The ONLY way to truly expand and evolve into your best version self is to deal with and heal the triggers that hold you back.

**You must become what you desire,**
**and healing is at the core of it all.**

Elevate who you are so you can get MORE of everything good out of life.

# MINDSET Shift 10

## Share Your Playbook

As I mentioned in the story about Phil, I shared something from my playbook. We have operators' manuals for everything except people, but what if we shared our personal playbook with others in our lives? How much better would this be for every relationship?

It's a pretty easy concept. But it does call for us to be vulnerable and transparent. People aren't mind readers, yet so often *we* expect them to be. And when we fail to be vulnerable, just like what happened with my friend Jenny, we get mad.

What is your playbook? Just like athletes have a playbook, or products have operators' manuals, so should we all. Your personal playbook is all of the ways you communicate best, and what you think others should know so that you can effectively communicate. It is everything you have learned in this book about emotional intelligence. It is all of the ways you hope to gain better self-awareness.

As we become more self-aware, we understand our **playbook** better. Sharing it saves so much time guessing, tap dancing, walking on eggshells, reading between the lines, and scratching our heads trying to figure each other out. Transparency and vulnerability are power, not weakness. We are all flawed human beings, ultimately wanting the same things: to be loved, adored, accepted and happy. That's nothing to be ashamed of. Accepting and embracing these principles are keys to getting MORE of everything good out of life.

## MINDSET Shift 11

### Forgiveness is Freedom

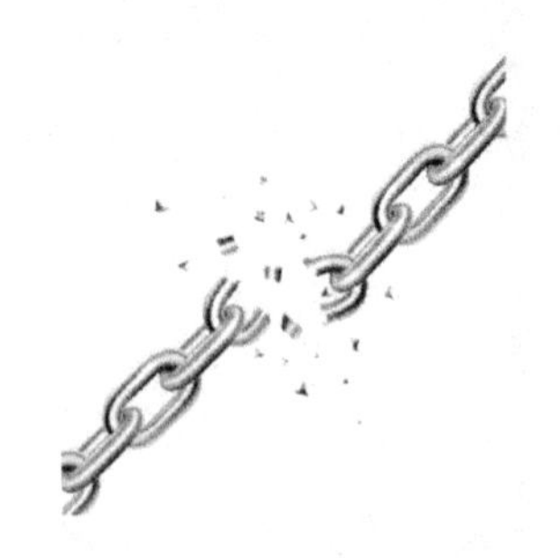

**FORGIVENESS**
**=**
**HAPPINESS**

Anger causes emotional unrest, and emotional unrest is linked to physical disease. Anger is a very low frequency emotion that attracts more low frequency people and circumstances in our lives.

Essentially, holding onto anger causes your own suffering. It's like drinking poison that causes unhappiness and adversely affects our well-being.

The irony is, the people at you are angry at usually don't even care that you are angry at all.

Anger gives the illusion of power. How many angry people have we seen in positions of power? How many red faces have graced boardroom tables under the guise of passion? How many friendships and families have been destroyed in the stubbornness of anger and needing to be right?

But when you hold on to anger, you are giving your power away to the person with whom you are angry. Is that what you really want to do?

Letting go of anger embraces all of the mindset shifts above. It brings *freedom* into your life. It creates more space for good, positive, high frequency people and experiences. It allows your energy to stay in an aligned place, therefore naturally making life easier. Letting go of anger makes you a magnet for other positive, productive people. If you encounter people who are always mad at someone, complaining about people, and essentially angry at the world, know that they are really unhappy inside. Keep those people at a distance; do not let their negative dialogues and energy bring you into their vortex of toxicity. If they are people who desire to change, model and guide them. But keep them at limited doses in your life if they are adversely affecting you until they make incremental improvements.

When we forgive, we create emotional freedom for ourselves to grow and flourish to more expansively than ever before. We also create the space for what I believe is the greatest achievement: **inner peace.** When we are consistently experiencing inner peace, we are undoubtedly getting MORE of everything good in life!

## Summary of the Shifts

These mindset shifts are incredible tools in your toolbox of living a more responsive versus reactive emotionally intelligent life. Write them down on a piece of paper and have them around you if you need to as you condition your new response patterns.

The more you use them, the MORE you will get what you desire in life.

## Journaling Prompts

1) In what situations do you frequently find yourself reacting rather than responding? How can you remind yourself to respond appropriately the next time you are in that situation?

2) In what ways can you prescribe positive meaning to the rest of the events you will experience today? How will you remind yourself to do so?

3) Think of at least three hurtful events from your past that still cause an emotional effect in you. How can you reframe them have a positive effect on your life? What lessons did these events teach you? What skills did they help you develop? How have they aided you in the long run?

4) Honestly answer the question, "Would you rather be right or happy?" Consider the question in light of your family, your friends, your work, and any other venues that are central to your life. How can you lessen the control that your ego has on your answer to that question?

5) What expectations do you have for others that you can either a) express to them now before conflict

arises or b) loosen your grip on to allow others the space to act based on their own experiences?

6) What conflicts are you avoiding right now that may be necessary for relational healing and growth?

## CHAPTER 6

# EXCEL

## In All Aspects of Life

**Everything is interconnected.**

**Everything.**

And as much as people would like to think it is possible to go through life putting our "stuff" into boxes, we really can't—at least not for a sustainable period of time before we see the adverse effects of it.

So, I am going to let you in on another secret. You are a human, not a robot.

We are humans! We have feelings and emotions, and the more we understand them and know how to process and harness them, the more powerful we can be.

Unfortunately, our societal norm is to ignore our feelings and emotions: to sweep them under the rug, brush them off, build our walls, shut down, and disconnect. How many times have you heard "men don't cry" or "buck up, buttercup!" Beliefs like these continue to create an extremely emotionally unavailable or unaware society, which perpetuates damage on others.

We cannot thrive when we are emotionally unavailable and in *shut down* mode. **The walls we create to keep us "safe" are actually the same walls that keep us from what we desire**. Sometimes we only build walls in certain aspects of our lives, like relationships, but these walls can still impact other aspects because everything is interconnected. On the flip side, the more we are open, emotionally available, and aware, the more we can deeply connect to ourselves and our purpose. When we do this, we get MORE out of life.

Holistic success is what we all should be striving for. In order to achieve holistic success, we must strive to become successful in all aspects of our lives, not just one or two.

There are four core interconnected quadrants in our lives that we constantly need to fuel.

- Health
- Finances
- Relationships
- Personal Evolution

If your health is poor, it will affect all of these other quadrants. If your finances are suffering, it will undoubtedly impact your health and relationships. If one (or more) of your key relationships is experiencing difficulty, it will surely impair your health as well as your ability to focus and be productive at work, which trickles down into your finances. You cannot compartmentalize these aspects of your life. It does not work.

If we acknowledge this interconnectedness, we become intentional in the way we live and nurture all of the aspects of our life regularly. As a result, we won't wake up one day and find everything out of balance or see things come crashing down around us.

To help build the intentional habit of assessing the four quadrants, become clear as to what your goals are for each quadrant. Write these goals down in your MORE Method Journal. Notice how each goal cross-references in the quadrants. You may recognize some conflicts among your quadrant goals, which means you will need to explore what beliefs or habits need to shift to help everything balance. Doing this exercise helps magnify what is important in all aspects of our lives, which also helps us shed the beliefs and behaviors that no longer serve us.

For example, you may write down a few big financial goals. Your belief system around money might be that you have to work more to make more money. But, at the same time in your relationship quadrant, one of your goals might be to spend more time with your family. Can you see the contradiction there? Since there are only so many hours in the day, your solution to work more in order to bring home the bacon will not work in meeting your relationship goals. This is where you will be pushed out of your comfort zone to get more creative and strategic. Instead, if you want to make more money but also want to spend more time with your family, you are going to need to create more passive income streams rather than just trying to get more money through dollars per hour model. Perhaps you solve both problems by investing in real estate or rental property or creating a consulting business. Whatever you decide at the moment may not yield the immediate results you desire, but the important part is you are moving in the right direction to achieve both goals.

The key lesson is that you cannot continue to do the same thing expecting different results. You must change things to change your results.

Some major questions in this scenario to ask yourself to find clarity are:

1) How can I improve my beliefs and means around making money?

**Maybe...**

- Create passive income/investment ideas and strategies
- Analyze existing talents and explore if there is a better career path for me
- Realize I am being undervalued where I am at work and ask for a raise, bonus, or new position
- Change my "work hard" mindset to a "work smart" mindset

2) How can I prioritize my days better to spend more quality time with my family?

**Maybe...**

- Wake up an hour earlier to get my workout done before everyone else wakes up

- Ask my boss to work from home some days to cut down on commute time
- Eliminate or cut down on TV time at night and use that time to get work done to leave the office earlier

3) How can I be more present with my family through activities? What are the top priorities and why?

**Maybe...**

- Sports Activities
- School Parties
- Vacation time
- Homework time

**As we begin to evaluate the microcosms of our lives, we can become more and more clear about how we spend our time and energy, why we do what we are doing, and what we need to change in order to achieve more and receive more. Self-reflection and life auditing exercises like this are really valuable to do frequently so we don't always default back to "auto-pilot".**

Here is another example: perhaps you notice your health and energy are suffering, and your top goal is to be healthier to improve your relationships, mental clarity, and financial/professional quadrant. You must first evaluate what you are doing to create your deteriorating health. Maybe you realize you have been doing way too much personally *and* professionally. You are the perpetual "yes" person because you feel bad saying no. If so, you need to evaluate a few things:

1) How can I get more *quality* rest?

**Maybe the answers lie in...**

- Going to bed earlier
- Having a better bedtime routine in place
- Watching less television
- Removing technology from the bedroom
- Taking supplements

2) What things am I doing that I really do not need to do, or can do more efficiently?

**Maybe I can...**

- Say no to events and parties I really don't want to go to

- Stop over-functioning for my children who can do things on their own

- Say no to committees at work that I was guilted into which really aren't benefiting me

- Delegate tasks that really do not need to be done by me both personally and professionally

3) What fuels me? What depletes me?

**Maybe...**

- I realize certain people drain me and minimize my time with them

- I realize watching personal development videos fires me up

- I realize certain foods are draining me so I eliminate them

- I realize I haven't been exercising and I know that makes me feel better, so I do it more

In becoming more aware of what new results we want, we can evaluate what is stopping us and make changes, creating new boundaries, new beliefs and habits, and get new results.

What also becomes clear is what we need to remove to meet our new goals, including the excuses we have kept using to keep ourselves small and a victim to our circumstances.

**Consistently nurturing and nourishing the four quadrants of our lives helps us life a more holistically successful life. The more we feel nourished instead of depleted, the MORE we can enjoy the many dimensions of our lives and get more of everything we desire.**

**NOTHING** in life is exclusive.
**EVERYTHING** is interconnected:

Your Health, Finances,
Relationships & Personal Growth

If one area of your life is suffering,
it affects the other areas.

Focus on all four pillars of your life
for optimal success and happiness.

## Journaling Prompts

1) Which of the four quadrants do you feel is suffering most in your life right now?

2) Building off of the previous question, how do you see the other three quadrants suffering because of the shortcomings of the quadrant you are most struggling with?

3) What habits make your body feel well-taken-care-of? Do you perform these habits consistently?

4) What would you consider the be your ideal, healthy, attainable financial situation? What steps do you need to take to reach that place?

5) Consider your relationships within your home, with your family, with your friends, and with your coworkers. How do you invest in those relationships? How do those people invest in your well-being?

6) How do your health, your finances, and your relationships impact your personal growth? Do they hinder you or set you free?

## CHAPTER 7

# TAKE **ACTION**

## Claim the Life You Desire

It's one thing to KNOW something; it is another thing to BE something. As I've said before, you must BECOME what it is you desire.

If you desire more high-quality relationships, you must be a high-quality person.

If you desire more abundance in your life, you must have an abundant mindset and act abundantly to yourself and others.

If you desire to have more contagious energy, you must think and behave like a high energy person.

I think you are getting the picture, right?

The difference between the people who will now live the life they desire and the ones who will not, are the ones who will take daily intentional action and commit to the changes needed to achieve what they desire. As I mentioned throughout this book, sometimes the small behavioral changes can heed big results. If you feel overwhelmed, then take small steps, regularly adding more small steps, to make big changes. Remember, **this isn't a path of perfection but a more conscious path to course-correct quickly when we make mistakes or see we are going off course.**

Now that you have read the previous chapters, reflected, and filled out your answers in the MORE Method Journal, I would love for you to go back to the original question in Chapter 2: "What do you want MORE of?" Did it change? Or did it remain the same? Often people will say they changed or added to what they originally had.

Now go into your MORE Method Journal and outline how you will get what you want MORE of.

What new habits will you start?

What beliefs will you change? What are some new affirmations you can create to reprogram from the old beliefs to the new beliefs (like I did for the beliefs I had around fear of failure)?

What behaviors will you minimize or eliminate to achieve your goals? For example, perhaps it's less time watching television? Or changing the type of people you surround yourself with? Or ceasing to eat poorly because it sabotages your energy?

What daily visualizations will you do? Align them with your goals and *feel* into them daily.

Who can you get to join you on this journey? Can they be your accountability partner(s)?

Having friends and accountability partners on your transformational journey is incredibly important.

What does your life look like one year from now? Three years from now?

How can you help teach others around you this information? How can you help elevate your family and friends so everyone around you can get MORE of everything good out of life? How will that make you feel to witness and be a part of? How can you make inspiring and empowering others around you part of your life mission?

What is your life mission/purpose?

I would love it if you would connect with me and share these answers and more by joining our

Facebook community https://www.facebook.com/TheMoreMethod/. In this Facebook group I will be sharing tips, information, encouragement, and much more as we continue to help UPLEVEL as many lives as possible, because no one should settle for a life of mediocrity.

I am so grateful to have had you on this journey with me. I appreciate your trust in me to guide you. I hope that the content I have shared has been impactful and as transformational for you as it was for me. My life's mission is to inspire and empower as many people as possible to know that they are capable and worth MORE than they ever thought was possible. Thank you for helping me live out my purpose.

## Journaling Prompts

1) What do you want MORE of now that you have finished this book? How has your answer evolved throughout the time you've been reading this and working through the journaling exercises?

2) What challenges do you anticipate facing as you adjust your actions to attain the life you desire? How will you overcome them?

3) What changes have you noticed in your life already as you've applied what you've learned while reading this book?

4) Who will you share this newfound knowledge with? What aspects of the MORE Method do you hope to share with your friends and family so they can also enjoy their best possible lives?

*Live your life with Passion & Purpose!*

"My mission is to **inspire** and **empower** as many people as possible to know they are **capable** and **worth more** than they ever thought possible."

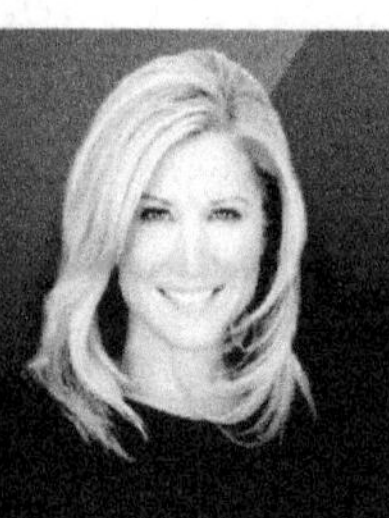

For coaching courses or booking
for speaking and training:

**www.jengroover.com**

@jengroover

@jengroover

@jengroover

@jengroover

## MORE Praise for

# The MORE Method

*Jen's teaching are life changing! I brought Jen in to work with my team over two years ago and we still utilize her MORE Method techniques today. It has had a tremendous positive impact on my teams professional and personal lives. We communicate more freely and have a deep understanding of each other's needs, desires and contributions. We also have a greater appreciation of why we may be behaving a certain way and how we can help. Jen's enthusiasm and passion for EI is genuine and clear with everything she does. This book will certainly transform people's lives.*

**Bill Emerson**

President, Emerson Group Inc.

*Before I connected with Jen Groover I was living in a comfort zone allowing life to just happen, being more reactive than proactive.*

*Since working with Jen and being introduced to The More Method, the trajectory of my life has changed. It has helped me to change my mindset and gain clarity by removing mental roadblocks and limiting beliefs that kept me from realizing my true potential in life. I have gone from dreaming to believing to actually doing things I never thought were possible in a short period of time. It's never too late to become a conscious creator of your life and to live with passion and purpose. Jen Groover and The More Method has given me the courage and tools to do so.*

**Donna Noga**
Head of Business Development Manager and Legal
Liaison, Delaware Orthopedic Specialists

*Jen's MORE Method has completely transformed my life. Prior to Jen, I was living in a world of wishes; wishing for more time, wishing for more financial freedom, wishing for a sense of fulfillment. Within one short week of practicing the MORE method I had shifted my mindset COMPLETELY – I started uncovering false beliefs, understanding my own emotions, pushing through my fears and even developing a whole new found love for myself. It is in this breakthrough that I was able to show up as the best version of myself – the best mother, the best wife, the best employee, the best friend, the best leader. The more I practiced the MORE method the more I started to feel alive; the more I woke up excited; the more I inspired the people around me. Before I knew it I had realized that while nothing in my outside world had changed, I had become the happiest version of myself. Jen taught me that BELIEVING means seeing, that alignment brings magical abundance and that you CAN accomplish anything. Thank you Jen for having such a profound impact on my life and for showing me the way to march towards a life of abundance. More importantly, thank you from my children who will only know a mother that operates from a place of courage, joy, and love.*

*Forever grateful,*

**Jen Martinelli**
Co-Founder & CEO Canvas Recruit

**Formerly unfulfilled employee wishing for more time, more financial freedom and a sense of fulfillment.**

Made in United States
North Haven, CT
21 January 2022